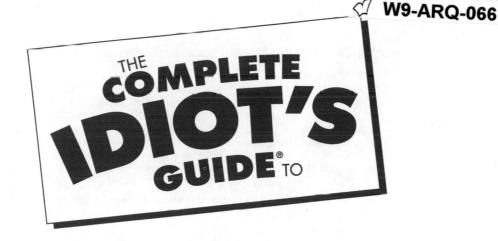

THE **COMPLETE IDIOT'S GUIDE®** TO

Wellness

by Patricia Burkhart Smith and
Muriel MacFarlane, R.N., M.A., with
Eugene Kalnitsky, M.D.

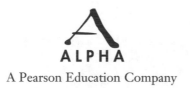

ALPHA

A Pearson Education Company

International Standard Book Number: 0-02-864343-7
Library of Congress Catalog Card Number: 2002103790

04   03   02   8   7   6   5   4   3   2   1

Interpretation of the printing code: The rightmost number of the first series of numbers is the year of the book's printing; the rightmost number of the second series of numbers is the number of the book's printing. For example, a printing code of 02-1 shows that the first printing occurred in 2002.

Printed in the United States of America

For marketing and publicity, please call: 317-581-3722

The publisher offers discounts on this book when ordered in quantity for bulk purchases and special sales.

For sales within the United States, please contact: Corporate and Government Sales, 1-800-382-3419 or corpsales@pearsontechgroup.com

Outside the United States, please contact: International Sales, 317-581-3793 or international@pearsontechgroup.com

Publisher: *Marie Butler-Knight*
Product Manager: *Phil Kitchel*
Managing Editor: *Jennifer Chisholm*
Acquisitions Editor: *Mike Sanders*
Development Editor: *Suzanne LeVert*
Senior Production Editor: *Christy Wagner*
Copy Editor: *Jeff Rose*
Illustrator: *Jody Schaeffer*
Cover/Book Designer: *Trina Wurst*
Indexer: *Ginny Bess*
Layout/Proofreading: *Becky Harmon, Mary Hunt, Brad Lenser*

Contents at a Glance

Appendixes

Contents

Foreword

At a time when the incidence of obesity and its associated illnesses are increasing dramatically for both adults and children, the concept of personal wellness is more necessary than ever before. But you shouldn't associate "wellness" with a simple lack of disease or injury. It's much more than that; wellness connotes the presence of vibrant good health.

We live in a busy, fast-paced society that creates unhealthy levels of stress and anxiety for many people. Our hectic pace leaves little time for exercise or for planning and preparing healthy meals and snacks. Neglecting the basic, essential needs of our bodies, minds, and spirits is a recipe for a decreased quality of life and potentially for developing debilitating or deadly illnesses.

Wellness is the joyous alternative to mere existence—to living with fatigue, a lack of energy and stamina, excess stress, and a high potential for illness. Living in a state of wellness has a positive impact on every aspect of your life: physical, mental, spiritual, and emotional health.

In addition to all the benefits that derive from including daily exercise, a healthy diet, and effective stress management into your wellness lifestyle, I just absolutely love the way being well makes me feel and the energy it gives me. There really is a stark difference between just the lack of disease and true wellness.

In *The Complete Idiot's Guide to Wellness*, Patricia Smith and Muriel MacFarlane have done a wonderful job of making wellness easy to understand and obtain. They've eliminated the complexity and provided an easy-to-follow, step-by-step guide to achieving wellness. While every aspect of the subject is well-covered, I especially liked the sections on planning meals and snacks, the importance of sleep, scheduling time to take care of yourself, and tracking your progress. As an exercise physiologist, I look at any information on exercise with a very critical eye, but the ideas presented in this book passed my litmus test with flying colors.

Congratulations, in your hands is a tool that can drastically change your life. Now get started!

Greg Landry, M.S., exercise physiologist

Introduction

As baby boomers began to enter their fourth, fifth, and sixth decades of life, popular American culture saw a surge of interest in the topic of wellness. Suddenly, after experiencing a few aches and pains or perhaps an illness or accident that landed them in the hospital, boomers wanted to learn how to stay well. Now, as the stresses of everyday life continue to escalate and people struggle to find ways to stay safe and sane in an increasingly crazy world, wellness interests everyone.

Walk into any bookstore and you will find the health section shelves lined with book after book offering advice about how to live with diabetes, heart disease, chronic fatigue syndrome, fibromyalgia, arthritis, and a host of other physical ailments. For a while we seemed to accept that aging automatically equaled deteriorating health. Now we know better. Now we know that wellness is a concept we can incorporate into our daily lives to help us stay healthy and happy, which, in turn, generally means we will live longer and more fulfilling lives.

Even practitioners of traditional or allopathic medicine are getting on the wellness bandwagon. Instead of waiting for people to get sick and repeatedly treating patients with a long list of physical and emotional problems, many modern doctors are finally turning their attention toward actively keeping people well. This is a welcome development.

The science of wellness is so new that the specialty is not yet formally recognized. Yet as we continue to develop tools and protocols to help individuals take control of their own health, it is our prediction that wellness will evolve into a full-blown medical specialty, just as pediatrics or orthopedics are recognized now.

Alternative health-care practitioners define wellness as an attempt to bring the mind and body together in harmony to create a peaceful, productive, and healthy life. This book incorporates that mind/body/spirit approach. It melds the best information and practices from the world of traditional or allopathic medicine with discoveries old and new from the world of holistic and other natural health-care practitioners to give you a complete and balanced guide to the principles of wellness.

Whether you are recovering from an illness or injury or simply looking for ways to stay well, this book can help. During our journey toward more vibrant health, we will examine the four pillars of wellness—nutrition, exercise, stress management, and preventive maintenance—and explore how they work together. We'll outline simple practices you can incorporate into your everyday life to help maintain vibrant good health and ward off the stress that can make you sick. Some ideas might be familiar, others are things you know but don't practice, and still others might seem a bit unusual. But all have been proven effective in order to be included here.

In Smith's 15 years as a medical reporter, MacFarlane's 20 years as a registered nurse and psychologist, and Kalnitsky's more than 30 years as a practicing physician, we have become increasingly interested in promoting the idea of wellness. The idea of keeping ourselves strong and vigorous well into our late adulthood prompted us to investigate the principles of wellness for ourselves. In *The Complete Idiot's Guide to Wellness*, we will share what we have learned in our personal quests to develop a workable wellness plan for our families and ourselves.

We will send you on your way with one of our favorite quotations from Chinese philosopher Lao-tzu: "A journey of a thousand miles begins with a single step." May this book be your first step toward a lifetime of wellness.

How to Use This Book

To make it easier for you to design a wellness plan that suits your lifestyle, this book is organized into six parts.

Part 1, "What Is Wellness?" defines the modern idea of wellness and discusses the history and evolution of the concept. Nutrition, exercise, stress management, and preventive maintenance—the four pillars of wellness the book encompasses—are touched on in this part. We finish up with the unavoidable truth that wellness is something you have to work at, but soften the blow by revealing all the wonderful benefits a wellness program will provide.

Part 2, "The First Pillar—Nutrition—You Really Are What You Eat," covers the importance of good nutrition in maintaining excellent health and provides an overview of current popular dietary fads. You'll learn about the body's building blocks—protein, fats, and carbohydrates—and how to determine the optimal balance of the three in your diet. We debunk refined sugar and junk food and show you how to plan healthy snacks and meals. Finally, we discuss vitamin and mineral supplementation and how to make sure you stay properly hydrated.

Part 3, "The Second Pillar—Exercise—Get Up and Move." Sure it's more fun to slug out in your recliner, but if you really want to stay well, you have to incorporate some form of regular exercise into your routine. Almost everyone can start an exercise program; staying on one is the tricky part. Here we give you lots of tips for getting started and staying on track, including how to find an exercise program that's just right for you.

Part 4, "The Third Pillar—Stress Management," presents an overview of research that proves stress can trigger poor physical and mental health. Through quizzes and guided imagery, you'll learn how to identify your own particular stress triggers, then choose tools and techniques to help defuse them. You'll learn how to create a serene atmosphere wherever you go and become an island of calm in the middle of any storm. Finally, we'll teach you how to get a good night's sleep, every night, without resorting to prescription drugs.

Part 5, "The Fourth Pillar—Preventive Maintenance," outlines the most important health indicators to monitor for signs of trouble and stresses that catching small problems early can prevent them from becoming big or even deadly problems later on. Here we provide "Wellness Watcher" charts to help you track your progress. You'll also find health checklists so you'll know when and how often to get certain diagnostic tests performed.

Part 6, "Wrapping It Up," offers encouragement to readers taking their first steps along the wellness path. It provides a series of "carrots" and "sticks" designed to appeal to different personality types and activities to help you get focused and get going. And don't even bother giving us your reasons for not following a wellness program; we've heard 'em all and we're not impressed. Get going. You deserve a healthy life, and your family and friends deserve a healthy you.

Extras

Extras offer little bits of information and insight in bite-size pieces, perfect to nibble on when you don't have time to read an entire chapter. They are presented as boxed sidebars to draw your attention.

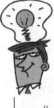
From the Medicine Chest
These boxes contain interesting anecdotes and tidbits of information to enlighten and amuse you as you start on the road to wellness.

Health Notes
Through the ages, people have had a lot of valuable things to say on the subject of health and wellness. Some of our favorites are included here.

911!
If you don't want to end up with a pulled groin muscle or in a perilous health situation, better read these warnings and follow their advice. They're meant to keep you out of trouble.

Wellness Words
No matter how much you know about health and wellness, you may stumble across an unfamiliar word or term as you read this book. They are defined here.

Acknowledgments

Writing is a solitary activity, but no writer I know can produce much that's worthwhile without the support of other people. I would first like to thank my wonderful family. My daughter, Meghan, and my son, Carter, have put up with a lot over the years just so their mom could be a full-time writer and wake up with a big, dumb grin on her face every morning. My amazing sisters and brother, Carol Stallings Edinger, Debi Burkhart, and Garry Burkhart, are always there to lend me an ear or a hand or a hundred bucks. The advice you all have given me over the years has been invaluable, but never as precious as your unwavering love and support. Finally, my beloved mom and dad, Nelson and Hugh Burkhart. Though you're no longer here in body, your spirits are with me always. You made me what I am.

I would also like to thank my editors, Mike Sanders and Suzanne LeVert. Mike gave me the opportunity to write this book, and Suzanne gave me a lot of support and advice throughout the writing process. A word of thanks also goes to the agent who put me together with Alpha Books, Sheree Bykovsky, and to Dr. Robert Moore, III, a friend and fellow author who took me to the Writers' Conference in Austin, Texas, where I met Sheree.

I especially want to thank Muriel McFarlane, R.N., M.A., for her contributions to this book. She rode to the rescue when an illness threatened to prevent me from completing the manuscript on time and did a terrific job writing the sections on exercise and preventive maintenance. Not only is she a skillful and accomplished writer, but it was a real pleasure working with her in what could have been difficult circumstances. I also appreciate the assistance provided by Dr. Eugene Kalnitsky, whose contributions were invaluable.

Last but certainly not least, I want to thank Chris Andretti, Trina Carpenter, and Christy Heiderscheit, who let me whine at them the whole time I was writing this book, and my dear friend, JacQuaeline St. Clair, who kept my house from turning into a complete sty as I raced to meet my publishing deadline.

—Patricia Burkhart Smith

My profound thanks to all my teachers, without whom it would have been impossible for me to learn and share the information presented here. Thanks to the many patients, who over the years helped me realize that lifestyle made a large difference in future wellness, and thanks to the publishers of all *The Complete Idiot's Guide's* who have made this easily read and informative book style so popular, thus making health information readily available and understandable to such a wide audience. Thanks also to my agent, Marilyn Allen, whose years of experience in publishing made my involvement in this project possible.

—Muriel MacFarlane, R.N., M.A.

I am indebted to my parents, whose sacrifices enabled me to obtain a medical education. I am grateful to my teachers, who gave me a sound scientific basis for the practice of medicine while inculcating that the practice of medicine was an art and that the secret to caring for patients was caring for people.

—Eugene Kalnitsky, M.D.

Trademarks

Part 1

What Is Wellness?

There seems to be something inherently unfair in the idea that the older we get, the harder we have to work to keep ourselves healthy and fit. Just when we want to curl up in our hammocks with a good book and a bad snack, our bodies are reminding us, sometimes none too gently, that we have to take care of ourselves. We can either fight it or we can get with the program.

The program is wellness, but many of us are not quite sure exactly what that word means. The good news is you can design your own wellness program, one that suits your schedule and temperament. The bad news is you actually have to do it to see results.

In these first few chapters, we introduce you to the concept and history of wellness and explain the four pillars that form the foundation of any effective fitness program. Yes, it's work, but it doesn't have to be hard work … it can be fun. That brings us to the incentive portion of Part 1. What's in it for you? Plenty. We'll lead you on with all sorts of carrots, so read on!

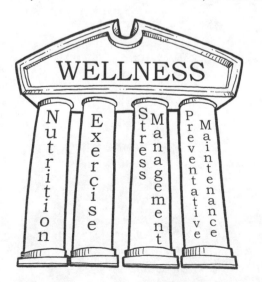

Chapter 1

Wellness Defined

In This Chapter

- What we mean by wellness
- But I'm not sick!
- What's your W.Q.? (wellness quotient)
- Setting wellness goals
- If you don't do tofu

Admit it. You wouldn't have bought this book and carried it all the way home if the concept of wellness didn't intrigue you at least a little. Even if you're the Beer and Pretzel King of Milwaukee or the president of the Couch Potatoes of America, Local Chapter Number 10275, you probably have at least some awareness of the state of your health. You might even be a competitive athlete or senior Olympics champion and still have some nagging worry that you could be doing more to help yourself stay well.

You *can* do more, and this book is designed to help you do just that. Achieving and maintaining wellness does not have to be an unpleasant task. Perhaps you're the sort who thinks that personal trainers are really medieval torturers in disguise and that professional dietitians should not be seen or heard. Fine. But you can still develop a beneficial wellness program that will produce significant results without submitting yourself to the tender mercies of a trainer or a food cop. Keep reading, and we might even let you spend some time on your beloved couch as part of your stress management routine.

Wellness Defined

Wellness is much more than just the opposite of illness. According to the *Merriam-Webster's Collegiate Dictionary*, *wellness* is "the quality or state of being in good health, especially as an actively sought goal." The word implies not only that you are *not* sick, but that you work at maintaining vibrant health.

Wellness Words

The American Heritage Dictionary, Fourth Edition, gets even more specific than *Merriam-Webster's* when defining **wellness**. It states that wellness is "the condition of good physical and mental health, especially when maintained by proper diet, exercise and habits."

There it is in black and white, straight from some of America's most eminent logophiles—you *do* have to work at wellness if you want to see and feel results. Wellness isn't just eating right or taking an occasional jog around the block. An effective wellness program should encompass dietary, exercise, stress management, and preventive maintenance strategies.

No matter what you may see on those late-night TV ads or read in the back of magazines, there is no "magic potion" or snake oil that will keep you feeling good forever. You can't just get a shot or take a pill to achieve wellness, and anyone who tells you that you can is probably trying to get his or her hands into your wallet.

Wellness Doesn't Just Happen

A few lucky souls are blessed with optimal health throughout their lives, but for most of us, wellness is not something that happens naturally. Most of us start out fairly healthy, but without an effective maintenance plan, wellness can gradually slip away with the passing of the years. Then one day we wake up and realize we don't feel very good, and we can't figure out what happened. Like any other desirable goal, we have to think about wellness and plan for it. Then we have to actively incorporate that plan into our daily lives.

Even if you suffer from an illness or chronic condition that prevents you from engaging in a typical wellness program, there are still things you can do to stabilize your condition and help yourself feel as well as possible. For example, people with arthritis who enroll in special P.A.C.E. (People with Arthritis Can Exercise) classes find the program not only helps with pain and stress management, but also increases their range of motion and slows the progression of their disease. Just be sure to consult with your health-care provider before you start any new exercise or nutritional program.

Modern Life Is Tough on Health

A state of continuing good physical and mental health cannot be achieved passively because the stressors that constantly work against wellness are not passive. Think about our modern world. Our bodies and minds are subjected to a relentless barrage of noise, traffic, pollution, toxins, and other extreme stresses that our ancestors never had to worry about. But there are positive steps we can take to allay the negative effects of these problems. We must first identify our particular stressors, then tackle them head-on with a well-thought-out game plan if we are to enjoy any measure of success. We can win the fight against injuries, illness, and the physical decline that can accompany aging as long as we realize we're in an ongoing battle.

You're Not Sick, but Are You Well?

Even people who are not actively sick may be walking around in less than optimal health. Chronic illness is particularly insidious.

The National Diabetes Clearing House says that at any given moment, there are more than five million people walking around with undiagnosed diabetes. A Johns Hopkins' study reports that there are an estimated 30 million Americans who suffer from undiagnosed high blood pressure. That means that for these two conditions alone, there more than 35 million people who don't ever really feel good, who are walking health time bombs.

We are all familiar with the famous high school biology story: If you put a frog in boiling water, it will jump right out, but if you put one in cold water and gradually heat it to boiling, the frog will stay put until it's too late.

It's the same way with sick people and the onset of illness. If we get very sick very quickly, we'll do something about it fast, but it is much more difficult to recognize an illness that sneaks up on us bit by bit. At first, we may recognize that something is not quite right, but dismiss it. We're too busy to notice, much less take time off from work or family responsibilities to go to the doctor.

Most of us get up every day, shower, perhaps get the kids off to school, go to work, come home, make dinner, do our chores, read a little, and then go to bed and start the process all over again. We're so overbooked we don't really have time to consider whether we feel good or not. As long as we're upright and breathing, we figure that's good enough and keep plowing ahead. But just because we don't feel "sick" doesn't mean we can ignore our health. That's how real problems start.

CAUTION

911!

Don't ignore early symptoms of illness and disease. Cure rates for Stage 1 cancers can approach 100 percent, while cure rates for late-stage cancers that have spread from their original site to other organs range from 5 to 10 percent. If you think something is wrong, go see your doctor. It could save your life.

Unfortunately, many illnesses get progressively worse if left unattended, and some, like cancer, hypertension, and kidney or heart disease, may even evolve from being highly treatable into something deadly.

According to the National Center for Health Statistics, at any given time, 1 in 10 Americans doesn't feel well, and that figure is higher among the poor (2 in 10). People who say they are not sick may really be saying they are not sick enough to slow down.

"Keep on Truckin'" May Not Be the Best Advice

How do you think colds and the flu spread from person to person? It's simple. People who are contagious and who should be home in bed heroically try to make it in to the office to finish that last report. When people who are sick with a communicable disease go to work or send their sick children to day care because they don't want to miss work, they jeopardize the health of others. A sick person in a social situation like an office or classroom may infect everyone they come near. Those they infect will then carry the bug with them wherever they go, spreading more misery.

From the Medicine Chest

Wash your hands regularly! From 1997 through 1998, Mary A. K. Ryan, M.D., a researcher with the Naval Health Research Center in San Diego, California, conducted an experiment with Naval recruits. After the recruits were ordered to wash their hands five times daily, Dr. Ryan discovered respiratory illnesses among the recruits decreased by 45 percent compared to the previous year.

Poor infection control and poor hygiene practices allow epidemics to get a foothold. According to Dr. Keiji Fukuda, a medical epidemiologist in the Influenza Branch at the Centers for Disease Control (CDC) in Atlanta, the flu kills more than 20,000 people annually in the United States and sends another 120,000 to the hospital. Yet it is difficult to get people to take a flu shot to protect their health against this known killer. We're more worried about exotic problems like Mad Cow Disease and Ebola, which have not yet touched our shores. If our culture focused on wellness instead of accepting illness and injuries as inevitable, we would all stay healthier.

We Know How to Be Sick

You don't have to be an M.D. to recognize when someone is under the weather. In fact, most of us would probably offer some expression of sympathy if a friend or co-worker exhibited a runny nose or other symptom of illness.

Our culture and our experiences have equipped us to handle illness. We've all been sick at one time or another, and we're indoctrinated with the right language and acceptable responses from an early age. We all know how to go to the doctor, take pills, stay in bed, rest, get plenty of fluids, and ask Mom or our significant other for chicken soup. A statement like, "That's a nasty cough; you should be home in bed" comes naturally, because seeing people with minor illnesses or injuries is fairly commonplace. But other than perhaps being told to wash our hands after we use the bathroom and before we eat, and to cover our mouths when we cough, how much wellness information was conveyed to us when we were growing up? Not much.

We Don't Know How to Be Well

How do we handle those rare souls who exhibit all the signs of radiant good health? What can we say? "Gee, Suzy, you're looking really, uh ... toned." Our language is hardly adequate, perhaps because the concept of wellness is constantly expanding and evolving and our ways of talking about the idea haven't kept up with its exponential growth.

Health Notes

The CDC says the top four ways to maintain good health are as follows:

- ◆ Eat a nutritious, balanced diet.
- ◆ Take regular moderate exercise.
- ◆ Do not smoke.
- ◆ Maintain a normal body weight.

Yet according to a survey published in the CDC's September 7, 2001, "Morbidity and Mortality Weekly Report," only 3 percent of the adult population practices all four of these habits. Women are twice as likely as men to follow this healthy regimen, with 4.5 percent of the adult female population as opposed to just 2 percent of the adult male population in compliance.

Many of us don't truly know what it feels like to enjoy exuberant good health, to be sound of mind and body. There are just so many things going on in our lives, so many problems that demand our attention, so many errands, details, bills, headaches ....

So What Does Wellness Look Like?

Though the concept of wellness may seem a bit hard to take in all at once, we do know it when we see it. A person who seems exceptionally put together and who is calm, confident, happy, and in control strikes us as the embodiment of wellness.

> **CAUTION**
>
> **911!**
>
> Do not undertake any wellness program without first consulting with your health-care provider to make sure the program you've designed or selected is appropriate for your needs and suitable for someone of your age and condition.

Wouldn't we all like to feel that way all the time? I know I would. But how do we get there from here, especially when "here" is so often a 40- or 50-year-old body that is weak, sluggish, too heavy, and nagging us with an assortment of aches and pains?

Where do you start? Start by figuring out where you are right now. Once you've identified your strengths and weaknesses, you'll be able to select a wellness program tailored to your individual needs.

Don't Know Much About W.Q.? Join the Club

W.Q. is your wellness quotient. You can determine yours by taking the following simple quiz. Your results are intended simply as a guide to get you started. Your individual program will vary according to the priorities you and your health-care practitioner determine.

Wellness Quiz

1. I am in my:
    a. Twenties (+0 points)
    b. Thirties (+1 points)
    c. Forties (+2 points)
    d. Fifties (+4 points)
    e. Sixties (+6 points)
    f. Seventies (+7 points)
    g. Eighties (+8 points)
    h. Nineties (+9 points)

2. I smoke:
    a. Yes (+30 points)
    b. No (+0 points)

3. I drink alcohol:
   a. No (+0 points)
   b. One drink a day (+5 points)
   c. Two drinks a day (+10 points)
   d. More than two drinks daily (+20 points)

4. I am overweight:
   a. No (+0 points)
   b. More than 10 pounds (+5 points)
   c. More than 20 pounds (+10 points)
   d. More than 30 pounds (+15 points)
   e. More than 50 pounds (+30 points)
   f. More than 75 pounds (+40 points)
   g. More than 100 pounds (+50 points)

   (Add an additional 10 points for every 25 pounds of additional weight you have over 100 pounds.)

5. I have a family history of heart disease:
   a. Yes (+20 points)
   b. No (+0 points)

6. I have high blood pressure:
   a. Greater than 140/90 (+20 points)
   b. Between 121/81 and 140/90 (+10 points)
   c. 120/80 or lower (+0 points)

7. I have high serum cholesterol:
   a. No (less than 200 mg/dL) (+0 points)
   b. Moderately high (200 to 239 mg/dL) (+15 points)
   c. High (240 mg/dL and above) (+30 points)

8. I have high LDL cholesterol:
   a. No (less than 100 mg/dL) (+0 points)
   b. No (100 to 129 mg/dL) (+2 points)
   c. Yes (130 to 159 mg/dL) (+5 points)

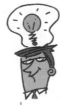

From the Medicine Chest

Our bodies actually manufacture cholesterol because it is a vital component in the formation of cell membranes, hormones, and other essential tissues. When we add too much cholesterol to our diets in the form of saturated fats from meats, poultry, eggs, and dairy products, we overload our systems and possibly start on the road to cardiovascular disease.

    d. Yes (160 to 189 mg/dL) (+10 points)

    e. Yes (190 mg/dL or more) (+20 points)

9. I have high blood sugar:

    a. Yes (more than 186 mg/dl) (+30 points)

    b. Moderate (127 to 185 mg/dl) (+15 points)

    b. No (less than 126 mg/dl) (+0 points)

10. I eat a diet high in saturated fat:

    a. No (+0 points)

    b. Yes (+25 points)

11. I eat three to five servings of vegetables daily (preferably fresh):

    a. Yes (+0 points)

    b. No (+5 points)

12. I eat two to four servings of fruit daily (preferably fresh):

    a. Yes (+0 points)

    b. No (+5 points)

13. I avoid sugary foods and simple carbohydrates:

    a. Yes (+0 points)

    b. No (+15 points)

14. I eat whole grains and cereals rather than refined:

    a. Yes (+0 points)

    b. No (+10 points)

15. I exercise regularly:

    a. Yes (+0 points)

    b. Sometimes (+5 points)

    c. Never (+20 points)

16. I get at least eight hours of sleep nightly:

    a. Yes (+0 points)

    b. 6 to 7 (+3 points)

    c. Less than 6 hours (+10 points)

    d. Less than 4 hours (+20 points)

17. I perceive my life as very stressful:

    a. Yes (+30 points)

    b. Somewhat (+15 points)

    c. No (+0 points)

Add your point totals and determine your wellness quotient using the following summary. Whether you've kept yourself in fairly good shape or let yourself get way out of shape, there are steps you can take to improve your wellness quotient.

0 to 30 points: You take pretty good care of yourself. Review the material in Parts 2 through 5 to see if there are any other strategies you can incorporate in your wellness program to help you maintain your good results.

31 to 50 points: You have a pretty good idea of what wellness is, but you're only human, and occasionally you fall off the wagon. Check your quiz results to determine your weak areas, then read Parts 2 through 5 to design a program that will keep you on track more consistently.

51 to 100 points: You are starting to get into an area where your lackadaisical approach to health could cause you some real problems in the future. Read Parts 2 through 5 and select a wellness program that suits your more relaxed approach.

More than 101 points: Your health habits are definitely putting you at risk for developing an illness or having an accident, perhaps in the near future. Read Parts 2 through 5, and make a commitment to yourself to make some serious changes in your lifestyle *before* you get sick or injured.

> **CAUTION**
>
> **911!**
>
> The National Sleep Foundation says that driving while sleep-deprived can be just as dangerous as driving while intoxicated. It slows reaction time, decreases awareness, and impairs judgment. If you are tired, avoid driving in the very early morning hours and early to mid-afternoon, because that's when drowsiness at the wheel is most likely to occur.

What Are Your Wellness Goals?

The first thing you must do before you get started is to determine why the idea of wellness interests you. This will help you write down a personal definition of the concept that has particular meaning and value for you. Why is this important? Because when you tailor your wellness program to your individual needs, likes, and dislikes, you will be more likely to stick with your program and be successful. Your own personal definition of wellness will help you set reasonable goals and figure out the steps you need to take to reach those goals. So let's begin.

From the Medicine Chest _____

According to the National Institutes of Health, here's what counts as "a drink":

◆ 12 ounces of beer, either regular or light

◆ 5 ounces of wine

◆ 1½ ounces of 80-proof whiskey

The NIH recommends that men limit their alcohol intake to two drinks per day, while women are advised to stop at one drink.

Why Does Wellness Interest You?

First, let's determine why you are interested in wellness. Read through the following scenarios and see which one applies to your situation.

◆ I'm getting older and starting to feel the effects of time and want to slow down the aging process.

◆ I feel stressed out and overwhelmed by my life and worry this might eventually make me sick.

◆ I'm still relatively young, in my 20s or 30s, and hope that adapting the principles of wellness into my life now will help me look and feel young for a longer time.

◆ I have a chronic illness and have reached the limits of what traditional medicine can do for me in terms of managing my illness and its symptoms.

◆ I've been ill, had surgery, or have been in an accident and would like to recover or improve my previous level of strength and energy as quickly as possible.

◆ No particular reason—I'm just curious because I've heard a lot about wellness lately.

Now read the recommendations that follow. They provide a good starting point for your wellness program.

I'm Getting Older and Starting to Feel the Effects of Time and Want to Slow Down the Aging Process

If you are interested in wellness because you want to slow down the aging process, welcome to the club. As the first wave of baby boomers began to enter middle age, their interest in the subject of wellness increased dramatically, and that interest spurred a tidal wave of sorts. In their quest to remain eternally youthful and fit, the boomers created a huge demand for nutritional supplements, more healthful foods, and exercise and health monitoring equipment. They bought almost any sort of book or tape they could get their hands on that contained information about health and fitness topics.

Here's your wellness strategy if you fall in this category.

- **Diet.** Plenty of fresh, leafy vegetables and complex carbohydrates to regulate digestion, balanced with high-quality proteins and a moderate fat intake. Avoid saturated fats, which can lead to heart disease, and sugary foods and simple carbohydrates, which can trigger adult-onset diabetes. If you have a tendency toward high blood pressure, moderate your salt intake.

- **Exercise.** Regular low-stress aerobic exercise like walking combined with moderate weight training to preserve muscle mass, strength, and bone density.

- **Stress management.** Hobbies, meditation, prayer, and volunteer work.

- **Preventive maintenance.** Follow the health checkup guidelines detailed in Part 5, "The Fourth Pillar—Preventive Maintenance," for your age category.

Health Notes

The U.S. Census Bureau says the population of older Americans has grown substantially in the last 100 years. In 1900, only 1 American in 25 was age 65 or older. By 1994, 1 in 8 Americans was a senior citizen. Declining fertility and mortality rates have led to a sharp rise in the median age of America's population, from 20 years old in 1860 to 34 years old in 1994. By the year 2050, the elderly population of America will have more than doubled to 80 million, meaning that 1 in 5 Americans will be 65 or older. But after the year 2030, the boom in the growth of the older population will slow down, because all the baby boomers will have already reached their golden years.

I Feel Stressed Out and Overwhelmed by My Life and Worry This Might Eventually Make Me Sick

The terrorist attacks of September 11, 2001, forever changed the way we Americans perceive our lives. Mental health practitioners reported an exponential increase in the number of people seeking counseling following those terrible events.

But even before September 11, modern life was pretty tough. Between working, caring for our families, financial pressures, traffic, and dealing with rebellious kids or difficult relatives or neighbors, it was difficult to find a peaceful moment.

You are wise to recognize that stress can cause serious and potentially fatal health problems, including cardiovascular disease, high blood pressure, and cerebrovascular events (stroke), to name a few. Your wellness strategies should include the following:

- **Diet.** Avoid coffee, tea, and any other foods or beverages that contain caffeine, which can increase your perception of your stress levels and make it difficult for you to fall asleep. To ease stress-related sleep problems, eat dairy and soy products, poultry, and whole grains, which all contain high levels of the sleep-inducing amino acid tryptophan.

◆ **Exercise.** Try exercises that burn a lot of calories like aerobics or jogging. Exercise for at least 30 minutes, and you'll trigger a release of calming and mood-enhancing endorphins.

◆ **Stress management.** Try meditation, prayer, aromatherapy, and/or deep breathing. For severe cases, your health-care professional may recommend a short course of anti-anxiety medication or tranquilizers.

◆ **Preventive maintenance.** Journaling is a very effective way to get a handle on stress. You might also try support groups. Get annual medical checkups to make sure your high stress is not creating physical problems, and follow the guidelines in Part 5 for your age category.

CAUTION 911!

Dr. Robert T. Scott, Ph.D., president of the Los Angeles County Psychological Association says: "We need to take stress seriously." Check out the following info and you'll see why.

◆ Three of the best-selling drugs in the country are used to treat stress-related illness.

◆ Eighty to ninety percent of all visits to health-care professionals are a result of stress-related illness and issues.

◆ Seventy percent of all accidents are stress-related.

I'm Still Relatively Young, in My Twenties or Thirties, and Hope That Adapting the Principles of Wellness into My Life Now Will Help Me Look and Feel Young for a Longer Time

Members of generation X and all the other upcoming generations have an advantage over the baby boomers in that they already know and understand the benefits offered by the wellness lifestyle. Follow these recommendations to incorporate wellness into your daily routine:

◆ **Diet.** Eat a balanced diet. Avoid foods that are high in saturated fats, sugar, and sodium. Eliminate artificial preservatives like hydrogenated oils.

◆ **Exercise.** Depending on your physical condition, vigorous team sports like basketball or volleyball can provide both exercise and social interaction. If you prefer to go it alone, try cycling, jogging, or strength training.

- **Stress management.** Try family outings and activities, meditation, prayer, journaling, Mom and Dad's Day Out, and support groups.

- **Preventive maintenance.** You don't require many tests, but some, like annual pap smears for women, are still essential. Follow the guidelines in Part 5 for your age category.

I Have a Chronic Illness and Have Reached the Limits of What Traditional Medicine Can Do for Me in Terms of Managing My Illness and Its Symptoms

The management of chronic illnesses like rheumatoid arthritis or lupus is one area where traditional or allopathic medicine falls short. People who suffer from a chronic condition often find they get better relief of their symptoms by combining the best of traditional medicine with the new ideas from holistic practitioners. If you suffer from a chronic condition, here are some basic wellness recommendations to get you started:

- **Diet.** It is well known that some foods exacerbate certain medical conditions. For example, red wine and other foods that stimulate the formation of uric acid crystals can cause an outbreak of gout. Research your condition and consult with your health-care practitioner to determine if there are certain foods you should avoid and others that may possibly offer some relief of your symptoms.

- **Exercise.** Many people with chronic conditions do not get any exercise, which is unfortunate, because exercise is helpful with pain management. Try a gentle form of exercise like water aerobics or search out special exercise classes for people with your condition.

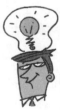

From the Medicine Chest

No matter what your condition, you can generally find a support group of people who suffer from the same condition. If you have access to the Internet, go to a search engine like google.com and enter the name of your condition in the search field. You will get back a list of links to information on your condition. If there is a support group available, its website will be provided.

By joining a support group or online community related to your condition, you will ensure that you stay abreast of the latest treatments and information, and you may even find that you are eligible to join a clinical trial to test new treatments and medications.

- **Stress management.** Try meditation and prayer. Join a support group with people who have your same condition. They can provide an invaluable source of knowledge and comfort.

◆ **Preventive maintenance.** Just because your condition is chronic may not mean it will be progressive. Work with your health-care practitioner to determine what steps you can take to slow the progress of your condition.

I've Been Ill, Had Surgery, or Have Been in an Accident and Would Like to Recover or Improve My Previous Level of Strength and Energy as Quickly as Possible

People who have just been through their first major illness or surgery seem to be particularly interested in the idea of wellness, but their condition may prevent them from undertaking a complete health and fitness makeover. The same is true of people who have suffered a disabling accident. One day you're your typical workaholic self, trying to cram 32 hours of work into a 24-hour day, and the next day, you are too sick or injured to move, or find yourself waking up from anesthesia. It can be a sobering experience.

If you fall into any of these three categories, your immediate need is for a wellness plan that will speed you on the road to recovery and prevent the development of additional complications that could make you sicker or further slow your recovery.

Many studies have shown that recovery from illness and/or surgery is appreciably faster when moderate exercise and good nutrition are incorporated into the recovery program. Here are some simple things you can do to help yourself recover more quickly:

◆ **Diet.** You need an excellent diet to provide your body with the nutrients it needs to heal. Unfortunately, excellent diets can be pretty difficult to come by in a hospital, home of the thrice-cooked wilting Veggie Bowl and Thursday Mystery Meat Extravaganza. Have a family member bring you cans of Boost or Ensure, or some other high-calorie, vitamin-, and mineral-fortified nutritional supplement. And yes, go ahead and eat the Veggie Bowl, if you can keep it down.

◆ **Exercise.** One of the most important postsurgical exercises is deep breathing, because lying flat for extended periods of time can cause fluid to accumulate in the lungs and lead to pneumonia. Hospitals use a device called a spirometer to help patients deeply inflate their lungs in the hours right after surgery. If you do not have a spirometer, take regular deep breaths that fully extend your lungs, abdomen, and diaphragm. Even if you are in pain, turning from one side to the other in bed stimulates circulation and helps to relieve pressure and the pooling of blood that may lead to the formation of bedsores. If you are able to raise your legs it is also helpful to perform simple leg and foot exercises. (Check with your doctor or attending nurse to make sure these are permissible.) Starting with your right leg, raise your knee and "draw circles" in the air with your big toe. Then raise both knees and pretend you are riding a bicycle. If you have had surgery on one leg, perform these exercises with the unaffected limb.

◆ **Stress management.** You're in bed, so enjoy it! When else will you ever have a chance to catch up on all your reading, watch awful TV programs, and get waited on hand and foot? Take advantage of this unique situation to rest and relax and allow your body to recuperate.

◆ **Preventive maintenance.** Ask your health-care practitioner to provide you with a list of things you can do to prevent a relapse or recurrence of your condition.

No Particular Reason—I'm Just Curious Because I've Heard a Lot About Wellness Lately

Now that you've read through all the categories, you may recognize yourself in one of them. If so, take a moment to go back, review the recommendations, and try to incorporate them into your life.

I Don't Want to Be a Health Nut

There was a time when people who paid very good attention to their health might have been considered a little nutty, but no longer. Wellness programs are sprouting up all over the place—at gyms, in outpatient clinics and hospitals, and even in churches. You can also find excellent wellness programs at many Fortune 500 companies whose top executives realize that it is cheaper to keep people well than it is to pay for their treatment once they are sick.

Indeed, corporate America is beginning to realize that helping their employees stay well is good business. When analysts studied GE Aircraft's 1992 employee medical claims, they discovered that claims submitted by employees who were members of the new company fitness center fell by 27 percent, while claims from nonmembers rose by 17 percent.

In a 1999 study, Travelers Insurance discovered that employees who were members of its fitness center took significantly fewer sick days than nonmembers. In the four years following the opening of the fitness center, sick leave was reduced by 19 percent.

Nevertheless, some of us have a tendency to look down our noses at people who frequent health food stores and gyms, who practice yoga and meditation, and who embrace simplicity. They seem to be the living, breathing embodiment of wellness as we know it today, but their very existence can induce guilt in those of us who love our ice cream and easy chairs.

But by buying this book, you've decided to take the plunge into wellness along with them. So let's get going.

The Least You Need to Know

- ◆ Wellness doesn't just happen; you have to work to maintain it.
- ◆ Being well not only adds years to your life; it also boosts your self-confidence.
- ◆ Even people who are recovering from an illness or surgery can follow a wellness program.
- ◆ Don't look at fit people as party-poopers; use them as inspiration to start your own wellness program.

Chapter 2

The History of Wellness

In This Chapter

- Wellness is nothing new
- Shamans and healers and witch doctors, oh my!
- The evolution of wellness
- Learning from the past

We wouldn't have such a wide-ranging appreciation of wellness today if it weren't for those early pioneers who paved the way before us, so let's examine how the concept of wellness has evolved through the ages.

We Didn't Invent Wellness

There's so much buzz surrounding the idea of wellness these days that we tend to think it's something we bright, smart, modern Americans thought up all by ourselves. Not so. The desire to remain strong and fit has been around practically since the dawn of time, though it did take mankind several centuries to figure out what to call that desire.

The word *wellness* dates back to 1654. The Middle Ages were a brutal time—if small pox or the plague didn't get you, then the hangman might. There must have been something about Oliver Cromwell's bloody reign as Lord Protector of the Commonwealth of Great Britain that turned one's thoughts to staying healthy, for it was then that the word *wellness* first made its way into our language.

Health Notes _____

The idea of wellness as an active life pursuit is nothing new. Way back around 90 C.E., the Roman satirist Juvenal (Decimus Junius Juvenalis) said it first and some might say, said it best: *"Mens sana in corpore sano,"* or *"A sound mind in a sound body."* In other words, almost 20 centuries ago, people who were concerned about maintaining their health already knew that it would take more than a simple pill or potion to keep them well.

Every Culture Has Had Its Own "Wellness" Programs

Though it took mankind almost 1,700 years to figure out a word to designate the idea of wellness, people had been concerned about their health for a long time before that word was created. Early pollen evidence from archaeological digs thousands of miles apart suggests that diverse cultures had similar knowledge of the healthful benefits of certain plants. More than two centuries ago, practitioners of *Traditional Chinese Medicine* (*TCM*) were already using acupuncture and herbal preparations to maintain and restore good health in their patients.

Wellness Words _____

Traditional Chinese Medicine (TCM) aims to restore and maintain the energy balance in the chi, or life force of the body. Practitioners believe illness results from stagnation in the flow of chi in the body, which prevents the body from draining fluids as it should. TCM includes acupuncture, herbal treatment, dietary therapy, and exercise.

Ancient Egyptian physicians advised their clients to wear cones of beeswax mixed with aromatic herbs and spices on their heads to ward off unwelcome and potentially dangerous insect bites. Mesopotamian herbal healers, also known as asus, prescribed bracing elixirs to restore their patients to good health. As part of a citywide sanitation system, Roman architects devised their famous aqueducts to carry fresh water into the Eternal City. Even in 600 B.C.E., they understood that maintaining basic standards of hygiene could help prevent illness.

The idea of wellness may not be new, but in a time of increasing stress and uncertainty, interest in the idea has certainly been renewed.

No One Likes to Get Sick

From the earliest days of mankind, when humans lived in caves and wore animal skins, to today, when we live in high-tech homes and wear designer clothes, we have suffered from a variety of injuries and ailments, frequently related to the environment. One thing that has remained constant since man learned to walk upright is that no one likes to get sick or hurt. If a modern breadwinner is out of commission, that circumstance puts his or her family in jeopardy. In the same fashion, the illness or injury of a senior tribe member, chieftain, warrior, or feudal lord would have had a devastating effect on the people who depended on his leadership skills to survive. We all like to stay well and feel strong and healthy, and that desire hasn't changed for thousands of years.

As a result, virtually every culture and society gradually developed various rituals, ceremonies, and other activities aimed at keeping its members safe and sound, or in other words— well. Some of these rituals were based on the rudimentary science of observation and employed various medical or hygienic practices to some benefit, while many others were rooted purely in superstition and had no real value other than psychological.

In addition to ceremony and ritual, as cultures developed and evolved they began to explore what medicinal plants and beneficial foods were available that might make them stronger and healthier. They began to understand it was better to stay well and whole than to try and recover from an illness or injury. This realization formed the foundation of wellness as we know it today.

Cavemen vs. Modern Men

We may think of our earliest ancestors as mere primitives and barbarians who could have nothing to teach us, but that wouldn't be exactly right. While the hazards of Neanderthal life were nothing to sneer at, modern humans face an even larger list of problems. You don't believe it? Let's make some comparisons.

Neanderthal Man	Modern Man
Extreme cold	Global warming
Animal attacks	Terrorist attacks
Vitamin deficiencies	Vitamin and mineral deficiencies
Seasonal malnutrition due to weather variations	Year-round malnutrition due to poor dietary habits
Food poisoning from spoiled meat	Food poisoning from new "super-bug" organisms
Clean air and water	Polluted air and water
Poor sanitation	Excellent sanitation in developed nations; poor in third-world nations
Lived an average of 35 years	Lives an average of more than 70 years

All right, so we don't have to sleep in caves, and blue jeans are certainly more comfortable than woolly mastodon breeches, but in some significant ways, we are not that much better off than our ancient ancestors. And in others, we are worse off. Cave men didn't have to worry about missing the five o'clock train or making their car payments on time.

Name Your Witch Doctor

If our ancestors hadn't been so interested in staying well, all those different tribes scattered across the face of the earth wouldn't have bothered to create the concept of a witch doctor or shaman. Throughout history, no matter what culture or era we study, we will always find some sort of healer that people turned to not only in times of sickness and injury, but also to brew up potions and spells to keep them well.

Today we have to contend with HMOs and PPOs, inaccurate bills, interminable waits, harried and hurried doctors and nurses, and ridiculously high medical bills. Before you start to feel too sorry for yourself, though, consider what some of our ancestors had to go through to get decent medical care. Even scarier is what some of the doctors had to go through if their treatments were not deemed successful.

Mesopotamian Doctors—Cure Me or Else!

There were two main types of Mesopotamian healers, the ashipu and the asu. The role of the ashipu was to diagnose the patient's problem by determining which god or demon had caused the illness or injury. It was sometimes decided that whatever was wrong was simply the result of some error or sin on the part of the patient. After making the diagnosis, the ashipu then performed charms and cast spells to drive out the offending spirit.

If this didn't work (and I'm sure you can imagine that it rarely did), the ashipu would then refer the patient to an asu, who specialized in herbal remedies. The asus were actually fairly skilled physicians. The world's oldest known surviving medical document, dating from 2100 B.C.E., describes the asu's technique for wound care: washing, bandaging, and making a plaster to cover the wound. That doesn't sound so very different from what we do today with our antibiotic ointments and Band-Aids. In fact, modern analysis of surviving Mesopotamian plaster recipes shows many ingredients possessed antibacterial properties.

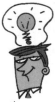

From the Medicine Chest

Pity the poor Mesopotamian surgeon. If he operated on a rich person and the patient died, his hand was cut off as a punishment for his failure. However, if he operated on a slave and the slave died, all he had to do was pay to replace the slave. Must have made it very difficult for the rich to find good medical care.

Walk Like an Egyptian

Like the Mesopotamians, ancient Egyptians believed that evil spirits caused illness, injuries, and death. The magical, the mystical, the practical, and the spiritual were entwined in Egyptian thinking. They also employed two different classes of healers:

- ◆ Magic physicians or "sau" were the first line of defense against illness. Often they were also priests. Sau were expected to figure out which demon was causing a patient's illness and then drive it out with magic spells and incantations.

- ◆ Lay physicians or "sunu" were often also scribes, the only people who could read or write. It was the sunu who concocted prescriptions and wrote them out for his patients. More than 800 "recipes" for sunu prescriptions have survived in the form of medical papyri.

Egyptian healers gave patients "prescriptions for a healthy life," which involved precise and regular purification rituals such as bathing and the removal of all facial and body hair. The distinctive black kohl eyeliner worn by both sexes actually protected against eye infections common in Egypt at that time. Healers also issued proclamations against the consumption of certain foods, such as raw fish and other animals considered unclean. Egyptians who adhered to this "purified life" expected to remain healthy as a reward. Those who didn't submitted themselves to dream analysis to find the cause of their illness.

Egyptians healers employed three distinct modes of therapy that have direct correlation to modern treatments:

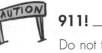 **911!**

Do not try this at home! In one ancient Egyptian prescription for birth control, the sunu recommends that women use crocodile dung. One can imagine that it worked very well.

- ◆ **Physiotherapy or massage.** Helped was restore usefulness to an injured limb.

- ◆ **Hydrotherapy.** Patients with orthopedic injuries often received a prescription for soothing warm-water baths.

- ◆ **Heliotherapy.** The Egyptians recognized that some ailments, like joint pain, responded well to heliotherapy or sun treatments. Patients were rubbed with scented oils, then positioned where the warm sunlight could soothe their aches and pains.

Ancient Egyptian doctors were highly skilled. Homer commented on their advanced capabilities in *The Odyssey*, and foreign sovereigns frequently sent for the best Egyptian physicians to treat their own families. They had particular expertise in treating and setting fractures, since many fractures occurred at the various pyramid and tomb construction sites. They also were profoundly knowledgeable about anatomy because of their practice of embalming dead bodies instead of burning them as many other ancient societies did.

In the area of wellness or preventive medicine, the ancient Egyptians reportedly fed their pyramid builders large quantities of garlic and onions to increase their endurance. They also followed one peculiar practice that is not so different from the modern practice of aromatherapy. They mixed aromatics like cinnamon and cloves with lard or beeswax and formed the mixture into cones, which they then placed on top of their heads. As the beeswax melted, the heavily scented wax masked any unpleasant odors that might have been in the air and uplifted its wearer with its enticing aroma. It also repelled biting and stinging insects that might carry disease.

Take Some Goat Cheese and Call Me in the Morning

The ancient Greeks studied Egyptian medical treatises and took them to heart. Their knowledge of anatomy was so extensive it even made it into their works of literature. In *The Illiad*, Homer describes almost 150 different battle wounds in great and anatomically accurate detail. Accurate descriptions notwithstanding, treatments still left something to be desired: When their surgeon, Machaon, son of the legendary physician Asclepius, was wounded in battle, his baffled fellow warriors gave him a cup of hot wine sprinkled with goat cheese and barley.

The Greek physician Hippocrates lived from 460 to 380 B.C.E. and is considered the father of modern medicine. He was a member of the cult of Asclepius, who was an ancient Greek physician who had been deified and lifted from mere mortal status to the status of a god because of his success in treating his patients. The healing temples or Asclepions that had been built by the cult throughout Greece were the earliest known hospitals. Hippocrates also created the *Hippocratic Oath*, which doctors still intone today.

Wellness Words

Hippocrates rejected sorcery and magical treatments for his patients, preferring instead to focus on treatments that had some scientific basis. Credited as the author of more than 60 medical treatises, he is most famous for authoring the **Hippocratic Oath,** a document pledging a reliable standard of care to patients. This famous oath became the foundation of modern Western medicine. In most translations, its first line reads "First, do no harm."

From this shaky start, Greek medicine developed rapidly, evolving as a mix of the scientific with the philosophic. They believed that human beings were part of the natural order of the cosmos and that any illness or injury represented an imbalance in this order. Their belief that wellness could be assured by maintaining balance is not so different from what many holistic practitioners believe today.

When in Rome ...

While the Greeks studied Egyptian medical treatises in depth, the Romans took a more relaxed approach to health care. In fact, the first doctor to come to Rome was Arcagathus, a Greek who arrived from the Peloponnese in 219 B.C.E. He was made a citizen of the Roman state, and in an early example of socialized medicine, the government underwrote the costs of building a medical clinic for the distinguished Greek physician. However, his vigorous and rarely successful use of the scalpel earned him the title of "the Executioner." His clinic was soon closed, and the good doctor was shown to the outskirts of town. An entrenched hostility toward the idea of introducing elements of Greek culture into Roman life prevented the further transfer of medical knowledge. There was also a sort of uprising against the mercenary nature of the medical profession because most doctors were rich. People preferred to rely on their own family members for healing and care.

It would be another hundred years before the idea of preventive medicine would rear its head again in the Roman Empire. In the meantime, Roman citizens relied on magic and lambswool, which they dipped into a variety of ingredients, for treating everything from bruises to lumbago.

One Step Forward, Ten Steps Back

After the relatively advanced thinking of the Egyptians and Greeks, medical treatment and wellness underwent almost a century-long slide, culminating in the abyss of the Middle Ages when the Black Plague swept across Europe, wiping out a third to half its population in less than two years. The plague spread rapidly because of overcrowding, substandard housing, and nonexistent sanitation.

Physicians who went from house to house to treat victims of the Black Plague wore masks with long, bird-like beaks filled with fragrant fresh flowers to protect them from the pervasive smell of death that filled the streets. Unfortunately, the actual culprits in the spread of the plague may have been hiding in the folds of their long woolen coats. It was not unusual for fleas to jump from the rats that hosted the *yersinia pestis* bacteria and carry the plague to human victims. The doctors who carried fleas with them as they made their rounds may have been spreading the very disease they were trying to cure.

Still, the Black Death resulted in some positive changes. The tragic epidemic spawned modern ideas of contagion, replacing the ancient idea that illness was due to some corruption of the sick person's spirit, and also led the Italian government to promulgate civil standards for sanitation.

The Rebirth

The Renaissance was much more than just a rebirth of the culture of a traumatized Europe, finally free after more than 200 years from the terrors of the plague. It was also the true beginning of modern medicine and health care, the time when ideas about wellness started to jell and evolve from mere folklore into actual practice. This is not to say that all was hunky-dory. "Surgeons" were actually barbers who pulled teeth without the benefit of anesthesia between haircuts and shaves. Public dissections became popular. The intimate knowledge the Egyptians had about the human body had been lost, and people were utterly ignorant about what was inside them and what purpose the jumble of organs and tissues served.

Still, most Medieval ideas about wellness and illness were rooted in ignorance. Physicians believed the body was made up of four equal parts of earth, wind, fire, and water, and they concocted many exotic, often painful, and frequently harmful preparations in their efforts to balance these four elements. It wasn't until surgeon Ambroise Pare discovered the importance of keeping wounds clean and how to tie off arteries that surgical knowledge started advancing.

Wellness Through the Ages

It's hard to think of primitive men being concerned with much else besides sheer survival, what with saber-toothed tigers and cave bears stalking their small tribes. They also had to contend with the onset of the Ice Age. Yet even among the early humans who lived more than 60,000 years ago, anthropologists have found some evidence of concern with health and disease prevention.

In the 1950s, Drs. Ralph and Rose Solecki discovered the remains of a 40-year-old Neanderthal man in Shanidar Cave in Iraq. While the other people in the cave were buried simply, the remains of this older man, Shanidar IV, were placed on a bed of woven woody horsetail and covered with flowers. Many of the other human remains in Shanidar Cave bore evidence of injuries, some severe, that had been healed. The older man's remains showed that he was possibly infirm and unable to care for himself. Yet his tribe had not only kept him around, hunted for him, fed him, and cared for him, but they buried him with great honor. Why? Anthropologists speculate it's because he was a shaman or tribal healer, someone skilled in the use of native plants as remedies for pain and infection, possibly someone who performed magic rituals to ward off evil spirits.

Although some scholars say this interpretation of the evidence found in Shanidar Cave is strictly speculative, six of the seven flowers found adorning this man's body have known medicinal and healing properties:

- **Yarrow.** Antipyretic, diuretic, astringent, and anti-inflammatory properties. Used to treat common colds and fevers, it is also useful against diarrhea and dysentery to control heavy bleeding and regulate blood pressure.

- **Mallow.** Laxative and anti-inflammatory properties. Used in poultices to reduce swelling and pain.

- **Grape hyacinth.** Diuretic and stimulant properties. Can also be used to make a primitive form of soap.

- **Woody horsetail.** Stimulant properties. Also useful for breaking up phlegm and treating coughs and respiratory disorders.

- **St. Barnaby's thistle.** Now considered a noxious weed that the U.S. Farm Service wants dead—they actually issued "Wanted" posters for it. Historically, St. Barnaby's thistle was prized for its lithontripic properties, or ability to break apart urinary stones.

- **Groundsel.** Diuretic, purgative, and anthelmintic properties. Used as a poultice to relieve stomach upsets and to get rid of intestinal parasites.

Only cornflowers have no known therapeutic value other than their beauty and pleasing scent.

Throughout history, people have alternately revered and reviled the men and women who treated their injuries and illnesses. If a shaman or witch doctor was successful, he was glorified, perhaps even elevated to the status of a deity. Unsuccessful healers often faced the risk of death. There is some evidence that the hysteria against "witches" that periodically erupted in Europe and even in America was perhaps due to a misunderstanding about the use of herbs and folk remedies. When a folk doctor, particularly a female, prescribed some brew and it worked, people frequently accused her of trafficking with the devil, because they didn't believe any mere mortal could effect a cure.

Those were dark times, indeed.

Today, our understanding of medical treatment and what it takes to remain healthy and strong is greater than ever. Yet we are still thirsty for more knowledge, for one more fact that might unlock the secret of perfect health and wellness for each of us.

With environmental pollutants increasing, our exposure to substances that could potentially cause illness is on the rise. Traffic, noise, financial concerns, relationship problems, uncertainty about worldwide tensions, even the biblical "wars and rumors of wars," all combine to create a level of day-to-day stress that is unprecedented in the history of man. Today, more than ever before, we need wellness to keep us sane and on track.

Lessons from History

Just because many of our ancestors' health practices seem barbaric by today's standards doesn't mean we can't learn anything from them. A careful study of the history of wellness and medical care provides perspective on the traditions we practice or reject today.

Despite a strong tradition of native healers and shamans, allopathic or traditional medicine has dominated health-care practices in America since the first Pilgrims landed at Plymouth Rock.

Allopathic medicine has provided many wonderful benefits. It's led to the virtual elimination of many deadly diseases, such as polio and tuberculosis, which used to decimate whole populations. And yet we intrinsically realize that something is missing from the impersonal ministrations of many traditional health-care providers, and that is the spiritual side of healing and wellness. In *The Complete Idiot's Guide to Wellness*, we'll combine the best of the old with the best of the new to provide you with a sound and practical way to take control of your own health and wellness. And we promise, there will be nothing in here that involves the use of leeches.

The Least You Need to Know

- ◆ The concept of wellness as an actively pursued goal is hundreds, if not thousands, of years old.
- ◆ Almost every ancient culture developed some sort of system to ensuring the health and safety of its people.
- ◆ Many ancient wellness practices still have validity today, such as the Roman idea of a sound mind in a sound body.
- ◆ The most effective wellness programs address physical, mental, and spiritual needs with a combination of sound ideas drawn from both the past and the present.

The Four Pillars of Wellness

In This Chapter

- A diet by any other name …
- Use it or lose it
- All stressed up and nowhere to go
- The importance of those 10,000-mile check-ups

Any balanced wellness program should incorporate nutrition, exercise, stress management, and preventive maintenance to be effective. We think of these elements as the four strong pillars that hold up your health.

As with anything balanced on four legs, if one of the legs is missing or weak, the whole structure may collapse. True wellness is achieved only by maintaining balance between the four pillars. If you exercise regularly but eat poorly and do nothing to manage your stress, you are setting yourself up for illness. If you eat right but never get up out of your easy chair, the same thing will happen. Even if you manage to eat well and exercise four times a week, the good benefits you accrue will not protect you from developing an illness if your life is full of unrelenting stress. Finally, if you do almost everything right but still don't get the recommended annual health screenings, you could let a little problem develop into something big and perhaps even life-threatening.

In the next few pages, we'll discuss each of the four pillars and how they work together to support your health.

Diet Is Not Just a Four-Letter Word

Simply say the word *diet*, and it's enough to make some people run screaming in the opposite direction. The very word seems wrong; it connotes deprivation and desperation. We all know that no one can stick to a diet for more than five minutes anyway, so what's the point?

The point is that more Americans than ever are overweight, and being overweight greatly increases the risk of developing a host of serious health problems. So how do we lose the excess weight? We go on a diet.

But the problem is that diets are no fun. If you're on a diet, you can't have that gooey chocolate fudge sundae with whipped cream, nuts, and a cherry on top that you've been dreaming about all day. And you can't have those chips and that giant 44-ounce soda. And forget about the extra slice of pie topped with ice cream.

Yes, we all hate diets, but a big part of the problem is the way we look at them. To begin with, we have the definition all wrong.

In its first definition of the noun, diet *Merriam-Webster's* doesn't mention a thing about starvation, deprivation, or missing out on all your favorite foods. It simply says, "a: food and drink regularly provided or consumed, b: habitual nourishment."

That's it. Our diet is our habitual way of eating.

It's not until diet becomes a verb that things get tough. There it says: "2: to cause to eat and drink sparingly or according to prescribed rules."

Now that sounds scary. Prescribed rules? Not at my dinner table.

Merriam-Webster's may have listed the noun's definition and usage first, but we would be willing to bet that if you asked 10 people on the street what "diet" meant, they would all give you some variation on the "eat and drink sparingly" scenario associated with the verb.

The word's etymology gives us some clues as to its original intended meaning. The Latin *diata* literally means "daily regimen," while its Greek antecedent, *diaita*, means "manner of living." So your diet is really nothing more than the habitual manner in which you feed yourself. And unless you habitually eat live bugs or some other such delicacy, that's not so scary.

Diet Is Not the Enemy

Before we even get to the comprehensive chapter on nutrition, we have a suggestion. Change your thinking. Don't think of a diet as a starvation regimen. Think of your diet as the fuel you put in your engine; the way *you* like to feed *yourself*. Close your eyes and remember that you are in charge of what you eat, no one else. And you can decide what goes into your mouth and what stays on the plate or in the baker's display case or on the grocery shelf.

Now that's empowering.

Out with the Old Thinking

I was raised in an era in which we could hardly sit down to a family meal without hearing some horror story about world hunger. Whenever any of us four kids dared to leave uneaten so much as a bite of food from our meal, my mother would launch into her "There are children starving in India" routine to shame us into swabbing our plates clean. We even had something at our house called "The Clean Plate Club." You could earn a little gold foil star on your chart if you finished all your food without prompting.

I have no idea why the idea of filling up my chart with those stars was so compelling, but it was. No sooner had my mother and father launched "The Clean Plate Club" than I was leading the pack. Modern parents couldn't get away with this tactic without promising video games, electric cars, and other massive prizes. But this was in the 1950s, when children were easily amused and distracted and occasionally even self-entertaining. Unlike many modern tykes, we feared authority, so when our mother or our father told us to eat every bite on our plates, we did, even if we had to choke the stuff down.

Health Notes

According to the U.S. Department of Agriculture, Americans annually consume 1,463 pounds of food per person, of which 624 pounds are animal products. This represents five times the annual food consumption per person in developing countries.

Childhood Memories May Control Our Ideas About Food

Fast forward a few decades, and you can see how dragging around all this guilt-inducing baggage concerning food could result in a few extra pounds. I had to really work at learning how to look at food in a way that was healthy and workable for me. I had to throw out all my old thinking and create a whole new way of looking at nutrition that had nothing to do with guilt or warm, fuzzy memories. I had to grow up.

It was especially difficult to overcome my childhood programming in the kitchen, where I worried that a celestial lightning bolt might strike me dead if I so much as left a grain of rice in a casserole dish. Now that I've freed myself from my old ways of thinking, I can actually dump leftovers in the trash without suffering agonies of guilt. That's not to say I waste food on purpose; simply that I know it will not imperil my immortal soul if I throw away a few scraps now and then.

Here's a quiz that might help you determine if some of your old ways of thinking about food may be preventing you from moving forward and creating a workable nutritional plan for yourself now.

1. When I was a child, my parents encouraged me to eat everything on my plate.
   a. Yes
   b. No

2. Mealtime was not very pleasant at my home when I was growing up.
   a. Yes
   b. No

3. My family usually didn't eat meals together.
   a. Yes
   b. No

4. When I was a child, I was allowed to eat lots of sweets.
   a. Yes
   b. No

5. My parents tried to force me to eat vegetables and other things I did not like.
   a. Yes
   b. No

6. My parents thought of me as a picky eater or thought I ate too much.
   a. Yes
   b. No

7. My parents or other family members made fun of my physical appearance or eating habits.
   a. Yes
   b. No

8. I used to sneak my favorite foods when no one was watching.
   a. Yes
   b. No

Count your yes answers and read your results.

0 to 2 yes answers: You have a pretty good handle on your nutritional thinking and haven't hauled much food baggage from your childhood into your adult life.

3 to 5 yes answers: You probably still hear your mother's voice inside your head whenever you reach for a Twinkie. You need to do some work to determine how you feel about food and nutrition and to figure out what really works best for you.

6 or more yes answers: You're dragging around a truckload of food baggage. Aren't you tired of letting ancient programming run your life? Don't you want to be in charge of how you think about food now? Yes? Then get going and do it.

We know a lot of this stuff is easier said than done, so don't hesitate to get help if you feel like you need outside assistance to rethink your relationship with food and nutrition. If you are simply confused about what to eat, a few visits with a registered dietitian may be sufficient to get you on the right track. The resolution of more complex problems like eating disorders will require professional help. You will not be able to maintain a new nutritional lifestyle until you have resolved all the underlying questions and conflicts that may have hindered you in the past. We will provide a comprehensive look at nutrition, the first pillar of wellness, in Part 2, "The First Pillar—Nutrition—You Really Are What You Eat."

Use It or Lose It

It is a function of the human condition that body parts not used regularly tend to diminish in size and strength over time. Although this may strike you as rather unfair, it is an inescapable fact of life.

Most of us can make it through our 20s and maybe even most of our 30s before our couch potato act catches up with us. But once we hit our 40s, things will literally go downhill unless we add some sort of regular exercise regimen to our weekly routines.

Those of you who are convinced that exercise doesn't have to be regular and ongoing to maintain benefits might be interested in the recently published results of a long-term study conducted by the School of Medicine at the University of California at San Diego. In the 1980s, researchers there observed 944 adults between the ages of 59 and 80 who regularly exercised three times a week. Using something called the BDI (Beck Depression Inventory), they discovered these study subjects had uniformly healthy, nondepressed attitudes.

When researchers went back to the same group of individuals in the 1990s, they were surprised to discover that the BDI for formerly upbeat people who had quit exercising had risen to the same level of depression as people in the control group who hadn't exercised at all over the 20-year span of the study.

The good news about exercise is that there are so many different programs available today that it is possible to find something to suit every personality and body type. Walking, jogging, swimming, cycling, kickboxing, yoga, tai chi, strength training—these are just a few of the many types of exercise programs offered in most communities.

The Motivation Factor

Just about everyone can start an exercise program; the acid test is staying on it for more than a few days. According to the Centers for Disease Control, 95 percent of the people who start an exercise program stop it within 4 weeks. The two primary reasons given for stopping are that the exercise caused pain and/or injury and the person could not see any physical changes or benefits resulting from the exercise.

Exercise, like nutrition, will not be effective if it's just a sometime thing. You have to figure out a way to make it a regular part of your life, a way that's going to work for you for the rest of your life.

Are you exercising because you want to lose weight, look better, be healthier? These are all worthwhile goals. However, if you are exercising because someone else is nagging you to do it, that greatly decreases your motivation and the chance that you will stick to the program in the long run. In order to be effective, an exercise program has to be something you choose for yourself because *you* want to look and feel better.

Which Exercise Will Work for You?

There are three main components in the selection of an exercise program:

1. The type of exercise you will perform
2. The length and frequency of your exercise
3. The intensity of your exercise

For example: "I will walk on my treadmill for 20 minutes 3 days a week at 60 percent of my target heart rate." This sentence includes all three components—type of exercise, walking; frequency of exercise, 3 times a week; and intensity of exercise, 60 percent of target heart rate.

Deciding which exercise to perform is more a matter of personality and preference than anything else, although it can also be a function of what programs are available in your area. Pick something that appeals to your sense of fun, and you will up the chances of sticking with the program.

The duration and intensity of your exercise is something you should discuss with your health-care provider or a certified personal trainer (CPT).

Aerobic or Anaerobic?

If you are beginning an exercise program, you will read and hear a lot of discussion about the benefits of *aerobic* versus *anaerobic* exercise.

Wellness Words _____

Aerobic exercise is any exercise that requires your heart and lungs to work harder to supply a sufficient amount of oxygen to your muscles. Examples include jogging and cycling. The clinical definition of aerobics is any exercise performed for at least 20 minutes while working at 60 to 80 percent of your target heart rate.

Anaerobic exercise is any exercise that requires more oxygen than your body can supply. Weight training is an example. Because your body tires quickly during anaerobic exercise, it requires rest periods between periods of anaerobic exercise to replenish its energy.

Each type of exercise has its benefits and its drawbacks. Most fitness experts believe programs that combine both types of exercise produce the best results.

Here are some benefits of aerobic exercise:

- Conditions the heart and lungs
- Helps control body fat
- Tones muscles
- Increases stamina
- Relieves stress and tension
- Improves mood and reduces depression and anxiety

You should be able to carry on a light conversation while you are performing aerobic exercise. If you don't have enough breath to talk while exercising, you are probably working too hard.

Some trainers recommend that you alternate aerobic exercise days with anaerobic exercise days, while others advise programs that call for 20 to 30 minutes of an aerobic activity followed by a half hour of anaerobic activity and then a cool-down period. Experiment with different schedules and combinations of activities until you find one that feels right for you.

Here are some benefits of anaerobic exercise:

- Increases muscle mass
- Increases strength
- Increases bone mass
- Increases endurance
- Increases resting metabolism (over a period of time)

Find Your Exercise Style

Before you select an exercise program, you need to ask yourself a few basic questions. Do you like to run in the great outdoors, or would you prefer walking on a treadmill in front of a TV set or while listening to music? Do you like to go to a gym to take aerobics classes, or would you rather pop an aerobics video into your VCR and exercise by yourself at home?

Here are some pointers to help you determine your exercise style:

Social exercisers:

- Like to exercise with a few friends or in larger groups or classes at health clubs
- Like to talk while exercising
- Choose exercises that will bring them into contact with other people
- May work with a personal trainer at a club

Solitary exercisers:

- Like to exercise by themselves
- Like to remain quiet while exercising
- Choose exercises that can be performed while alone
- Avoid exercise classes and personal trainers; prefer to receive exercise instruction from books and videotapes

Once you determine your exercise style, you'll find it easier to select an exercise program that meets your needs.

Fools Rush In

One of the most frequent reasons people give for falling off the exercise wagon is that their muscles hurt and they are too sore to continue. Anyone who's ever been around a football coach is familiar with the old adage, "No pain, no gain." Just the opposite is true of long-term exercise programs—if you've got pain, you'll lose your gain. If you dive right into an intensive exercise program without proper warm-ups before and cool-downs after exercising, the likelihood is high that you will suffer a buildup of lactic acid in your muscle. It is this buildup that makes muscles feel sore; the more lactic acid you have in your muscles, the more you will hurt. So if you want to avoid those postexercise aches and pains, warm up, start slowly, and don't overdo the intensity of your exercise. One way you can combat this buildup is to drink plenty of water, which serves to help flush lactic acid out of your muscle tissues.

No one is going to keep doing something that makes them feel bad, no matter how convinced they are that it's good for them. Remember, a good exercise program starts slowly and gradually builds in intensity and duration as the person's strength and endurance increase. A good exercise program does not make you feel like you got hit by a Mack truck. If yours does, something is wrong.

Don't Make It Burn, Baby

In the 1970s and 1980s, when we were first discovering aerobic exercise, a lot of exercise gurus used to holler, "Make it burn, baby!" Their whole idea was that any exercise that didn't make you feel like your whole body was on fire was no good. Today we know the exact opposite is true. Exercising with the intensity that was advocated in the early days of the aerobic movement led to a lot of injuries—some of them fairly serious. If you want long-lasting results from your exercise program, take your time, start slowly, and build gradually.

Did you get out of shape overnight? No, you did not. So why do you think you can sprinkle some fairy dust around, click your heels together three times, and somehow magically have your old body and endurance back? It just doesn't work that way.

If you want to see long-term results, you have to put in some long-term exercise. Get your body up and moving and stick with it no matter what and one day, a year or so down the road, you'll wake up and look in the mirror and your old body and strength level *will* be back. And when that happens, months of hard work aside, it will seem like magic.

For a complete look at exercise, the second pillar of wellness, see Part 3, "The Second Pillar—Exercise—Get Up and Move."

Tied Up in Knots

Modern life isn't easy. No matter what your age, occupation, or social status, day-to-day living is going to bring its share of problems and upheavals your way.

It's an undisputed fact that stress can kill, but it's not realistic to think you can keep every bit of stress out of your life. What you can do is learn how to manage your stress so that it is not so detrimental to you and to your health.

According to a 1993 study performed by Gale Research, the top 10 stressful life events are as follows:

◆ Death of spouse

◆ Divorce

◆ Marital separation

- Jail term or death of close family member
- Personal injury or illness
- Marriage
- Loss of job due to termination
- Marital reconciliation or retirement
- Pregnancy
- Change in financial state

If you've experienced one or more of these 10 events in your life recently, you should be especially aware of your increased chance for developing a stress-related illness. Assess your level of risk and take whatever steps are necessary to effectively manage your stress and protect yourself from its potentially harmful effects.

Is Stress Always Bad?

We have come to associate the word *stress* with negative events, but not all stress is bad. In fact, any unabridged dictionary should list two separate words for stress: *eustress*, or good stress, and *distress*, or bad stress.

In his 1956 classic, *Stress and Distress*, physiologist Hans Seyle, widely considered to be the founder of the theory of stress, wrote the now commonly accepted clinical definition of the word. Seyle said: "Stress is the nonspecific response of an organism to any pressure or demand."

Seyle defined eustress as the pleasurable emotion that accompanies feelings of success, fulfillment, and accomplishment, while distress is the emotion triggered by any negative event or feeling. Seyle was one of the first to note the relationship between stress and a negative long-term impact on physical health.

Top athletes and business executives frequently use feelings of anticipation and excitement to enhance performance at important competitions or meetings. However, like any good thing, you can have too much eustress. If that happens, those positive feelings might devolve into butterflies in your stomach or nervous dread. The key is learning how to keep eustress in balance so that it doesn't become distress.

Fight or Flight?

You may have heard of something called the "fight or flight" response. Put simply, this is the body's natural response to threatening situations. While it served our ancestors well, giving them the extra surge of energy they needed to outrun a predatory animal or battle their way out of a dangerous situation, today the response has become a health threat.

Our exposure to stress keeps increasing while our response to that exposure remains the same—we fight whatever is threatening us or we run away from it. In these situations, our brains put our bodies on the highest level of alert and starts flooding our bloodstreams with the stress hormones adrenaline and cortisol. The body responds to this hormonal stimulus by making the heart beat faster. Your muscles tense and endorphins and other natural pain-diminishing and performance-enhancing compounds are released into your bloodstream.

It is not good for your body to be awash in these powerful hormones and chemicals 5, 10, or 15 times a day. But think about your typical workday or an average day at home with the kids, and you will know that you feel the fight or flight urge several times in each 24-hour period.

What can you do to diminish your body's automatic reaction to stressors both major and minor? You can learn how to manage that response so that it works in your favor.

The Signs of Stress

Stress manifests itself in different ways in different people. Read through this list to see if any of the symptoms sound familiar.

Physical signs:

◆ Difficulty falling asleep or staying asleep

◆ Digestive upsets, nausea, bloating, cramping, and diarrhea

◆ Racing heart

◆ Tension or migraine headaches

◆ A feeling of tightness in the chest

◆ Generalized body aches or backache

◆ Unusual fatigue

◆ Change in eating habits

Emotional or psychological signs:

◆ A racing mind or the inability to settle down and concentrate

◆ Forgetfulness

◆ Paranoid or illogical thinking

◆ Irritable or easily distracted

◆ Impatient

◆ Unusually depressed or anxious

- Easily angered
- Feelings of isolation and loneliness
- Increase in use of alcohol and tobacco products
- Inappropriate use of prescription or over-the-counter drugs
- Use of illicit drugs

If you are experiencing three or more of these symptoms, it's an indication that your stress is reaching an unhealthy level and you need to do something to get it back under control.

Look for more information about stress management, the third pillar of wellness, in Part 4, "The Third Pillar—Stress Management."

Ten Ounces of Prevention

The last pillar of wellness may not seem as important as the other three, but it is. Even though preventive maintenance can be accomplished in most cases with an annual check-up supplemented by monthly personal exams and symptom checks, its value to catch and treat certain diseases before they get out of control cannot be overstated.

The particular tests and check-ups you need will vary according to your age and gender. As you move through the decades of your life, they will change to address the fact that the incidence of certain diseases, such as diabetes and cardiovascular disease, tends to increase with advancing age.

In addition to getting the suggested annual check-ups and diagnostic tests, there are certain symptoms you should watch for, because the development of these signs could mean your health is at risk.

To read more on preventive maintenance, the fourth pillar of wellness, see Part 5, "The Fourth Pillar—Preventive Medicine."

The Least You Need to Know

- Wellness rests upon four strong pillars: nutrition, exercise, stress management, and preventive maintenance.
- You should think of a diet simply as the way you habitually feed yourself, not as some starvation program.
- The best exercise programs combine aerobic with anaerobic activities.
- Stress management is one of the most effective tools you can use to enhance your health.
- Preventive maintenance is a vital component of any wellness program.

Chapter 4

What's in It for Me?

In This Chapter

- ◆ The benefits of the wellness lifestyle
- ◆ A sound mind
- ◆ A healthy body
- ◆ A renewed spirit

Before you start your journey to wellness, take a few minutes to think about exactly what you hope to accomplish. Do you want to lose weight? Lower your blood pressure? Feel better? Have more energy? Get a handle on your stress level? Sleep soundly? Establish more satisfying relationships with your family and friends? Boost your career?

You can do all this and more once you get on the wellness track. Determining your personal priorities and objectives will help you design the wellness program that will be most effective for you.

Living the Wellness Lifestyle

It's human nature to weigh potential results before we start something new. It's part of our decision-making process. When we embark on the wellness lifestyle, we naturally want to know what benefits we can expect for our investment of time and effort.

Wellness benefits accrue in direct proportion to the investments we make. If we decide to exercise five mornings a week but only manage to exercise three mornings, we will get a different result than if we exercised five mornings a week. If we don't stick to our plan at all, we'll get yet another result.

Behavioral scientists have developed something called the Transtheorectical Model to explain the steps human beings go through to change their behaviors. We'll use wellness to illustrate the five steps in the model:

1. **Precontemplation or ignorance.** You don't even know that the concept of wellness as an actively pursued goal exists.

2. **Contemplation or learning.** You've heard about wellness, and you are starting to think about whether it is something that might be of benefit to you.

3. **Preparation or planning.** You've made the decision to incorporate new wellness behaviors into your lifestyle and are starting to develop plans to make this happen.

4. **Action or doing.** You actually start incorporating new wellness behaviors into your life.

5. **Maintenance or habit.** Your wellness behaviors have become habitual, and you do them all the time without even thinking about them.

Obviously, the goal for incorporating any new behavior into your life is to stick with it until you reach step five and it becomes a habit.

The real trick is to keep practicing the wanted behavior until it becomes second nature. Think about your bedtime rituals. Maybe you brush your teeth, wash your face, change into your pajamas, and then fall into bed. How much effort would it take for you to add an additional 15 minutes to this routine? Just 15 minutes would give you time to reflect on your day, celebrate your successes, bless your failures, record a few observations in a journal, and spend a few moments breathing deeply and quieting your mind in preparation for sleep. Incorporating this new wellness behavior would not only help you to sleep better but would give you a private moment of sanctuary you could look forward to at the end of each day. No matter what happened during the day, you would know that you'd have the opportunity to look at it in a calm and rational fashion in the time you have set aside for yourself.

Change Your Habits, Change Your Life

The geniuses who thought up the Transtheorectical Model for change particularly emphasized the importance of going slowly and only tackling one thing at a time. A big reason people fail when they try to make changes in their lifestyle is that they want to change too many things at once. If you want to lose weight, start exercising, get to bed earlier, read more, and keep your checkbook balanced, that's all fine, but if you try to tackle all these projects at once your chance of success will be slim.

To make your master plan, you do need to identify all the areas you wish to change. Then you need to prioritize the changes from most to least important. Once all that's done, you can start to work on the most important one first. When you've practiced those changes enough to make them a habit, then you're ready to start changing another behavior.

From the Medicine Chest

Experts say that it takes 21 days to either break a bad habit or incorporate a new beneficial habit into your life. To increase your chances of success in eliminating an old, undesirable habit, try replacing it with a healthier habit instead. For example, if you're used to eating a big dish of ice cream every night before bed and you simply try to eliminate the habit cold turkey, chances are that you will fall off the wagon after a few days. One night, you might suddenly feel so overwhelmed with feelings of deprivation that you dive face-first into a vat of ice cream. If however, you replace the ice cream with a frozen fruit bar or low-fat frozen yogurt, you have a much better chance of eliminating the bad habit altogether.

Once you replace a bad habit with a less bad habit, you can work on refining the habit in incremental steps until you reach your final goal.

Write It Down

One of the most important things you can do to boost your chances of success when setting goals, trying to break bad habits, or incorporating beneficial habits into your lifestyle is to write it down. Use positive, specific language to describe the desired change. The simple act of writing down your goals does several things:

♦ It defines the goal clearly.

♦ It allows you to keep track of your progress toward reaching the goal.

♦ It allows you to keep track of the time you have been working on the goal (remember that it takes 21 days to break or form a habit).

Remember the Downside

Think about a typical day in your life. You probably awaken early, rush to shower and dress, and perhaps skip breakfast because you're running late. Heaven forbid you should take an hour out of your already jam-packed schedule to exercise, meditate, or write a few thoughts down in a journal.

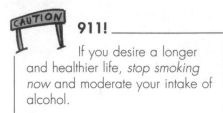

911!

If you desire a longer and healthier life, *stop smoking now* and moderate your intake of alcohol.

Does this sound like you? If it does, you are on the path to disaster. It may not happen tomorrow or even next week, but sooner or later neglecting the needs of your body, mind, and spirit will exact a toll on your health. It may be something minor or something more significant, but the odds say it will happen.

We presume you picked up this book because you care about the quality of your life and want to make it better. If you're tired of feeling harried and hurried and want to make some positive changes, you are an ideal candidate for a wellness program.

What Benefits Can I Expect?

The list is long, but here are a few of the most important areas where you will see improvement once you start on a comprehensive wellness program:

- ◆ Your physical health will improve in measurable ways—lower blood pressure, weight loss, fewer headaches, and improved strength and stamina to name just a few.
- ◆ You will feel less stressed and better able to cope with whatever pressures come your way.
- ◆ Your spirit will feel renewed; you will feel more positive and empowered.
- ◆ Your relationships and perhaps even your career will improve as a result of your more positive outlook.

These are just a few of the many wonderful benefits you will start to experience as you begin to incorporate wellness strategies into your day-to-day life. Not everything will happen all at once; some benefits, particularly in the area of strength and stamina, may require months to be fully realized. The important thing is to keep going; don't quit just because you don't see instant results.

It All Starts in Our Heads

So why is it so important for us to feel in control of our own lives and destinies? Because just about everything that happens to us starts inside our heads. Every dream, every idea, every worry, every fear—our own conscious and unconscious psychic energy makes them all become reality or prevents them from becoming a reality. It's really all up to us.

Dozens of modern motivational speakers have talked about the often overlooked power of our words and thoughts. There's not a book on the subject that doesn't advise us to clean up our thought processes.

If we are always poor mouthing, talking about how broke we are and how nothing good ever happens to us, then somehow that is the reality we manage to create for ourselves. Our brains listen to the messages on the subconscious tape that's looping over and over again in the back of our minds, and we make whatever is on the tape become our reality, good or bad.

Conversely, if we identify our highest goals and make a conscious effort to project those desires out into the world in a positive way, then we are taking a giant step in the direction of making those goals a reality.

Try this exercise. Stand in right in front of a mirror and look yourself in the eye. Now repeat: "*I* am in charge of my own life, no one else." Say it as many times as it takes for you to start believing it. Why is this so important? Because if you believe that someone else has power over you, then you feel helpless. If you feel helpless, then you arc at the mercy of life's vagaries and subject to all sorts of indignities over which you feel like you have no control.

How would you rather feel? Calm and in control of your own life? Or helpless and out of control?

See? Taking control is empowering. But remember the only life you can control is your own. Start trying to take control of someone else's life and you've opened up a whole new set of problems. Concentrate on taking care of you.

Taking Control Is Empowering

One of the worst places any of us can be in is to have a lot of responsibility with little authority. This can happen in a job where a middle manager is expected to get all the work done in a very short period of time but is not given the resources required to meet the deadline. Or a husband might expect his wife to run a perfect household and set a sumptuous table on $10 a week. Situations like this are real stress builders.

No matter how we may interpret whatever situation we find ourselves in, the bottom line is that we are the authority in our own lives. The proverbial buck stops with us. So if we are unhappy with our weight, our mindset, our careers, the way we eat, the way we treat other people, or get treated by others, we don't have to ask anyone for permission to make important changes. We simply have to decide what we want to do and then, as the TV commercial says, "Just do it."

Practice Positive Thinking

No one can argue that there aren't many terrible things happening in the world today; we've all seen the television pictures and read the newspapers. The trick is to not let the fear and uncertainty that governs the modern world rule our lives. If we wallow in the breaking news and never take our heads out of the first section of the newspaper, we run the risk of losing sight of a very important fact—life can be pretty wonderful if we just let it.

Oprah Winfrey has become famous for many things, but one piece of advice she gives seems particularly useful and relevant in times like these—she recommends that her viewers start a "Gratitude Journal," a place to write down at least one thing every day for which they are grateful.

It may seem hokey, but the simple act of gratitude helps us focus on the things that truly matter—our families, friends, health, homes, neighborhoods, and communities. Keeping a Gratitude Journal puts us in touch with the bounty and blessings of our daily lives, something that can get lost in the frantic shuffle of modern living. Another benefit: Making a daily thanksgiving part of our regular routines can serve to remind us just how lucky we are, which, in turn, insulates us from some of life's harsher realities.

Look Out for the Agents Provocateur

If there's one cliché about the human race that rings true, it's this one: "Misery loves company." If you hang out around the water cooler with the same three guys every coffee break, sucking down donuts and danish with a coffee or soda chaser while you complain about everything from the weather to your boss, don't expect these people to be happy when you show up with your bottled water and carrot sticks. No, they will more than likely don their black cloaks and become *agents provocateur*.

Wellness Words

An **agent provocateur** is one employed to associate with suspected persons and pretend sympathy with their aims to incite them to some incriminating action.

We use the term agent provocateur rather than saboteur here for a distinct reason. The dictionary defines sabotage as "deliberate subversion, destructive or obstructive action." Your friends wish you well; they do not deliberately intend to harm you or derail you from your wellness track. Therefore, when they wave that warm donut in front of your face, they are acting as agents provocateur rather than saboteurs. It's a matter of intent. They don't want to blow up your program as much as they want to entice you off your program and back into the donut corral with them.

Raining on Your Parade

People who are wallowing in bad habits do not like to see anyone else, particularly someone they know, pick themselves up out of the morass and make changes for the better. It makes them feel bad because it forces them to examine their own behaviors—something that is rarely a fun thing to do. If you have started on a wellness program, your former partners in coffee break crime will most certainly regard you as a "suspected person" and unconsciously do everything in their power to lure you back into the fold. When you momentarily lose your resolve (and every once in a while you will) and treat them to the spectacle of you shoving that four-pound bagel down your throat in two bites, it momentarily reassures them that their own bad habits are maybe not so bad.

The very people you might hope would be your biggest allies in your efforts to change may, in fact, be unwitting enemy agents always looking to undermine your success with a well-placed barb. Just be aware that they are out there and ignore them. Don't take it personally because this sort of behavior rarely is personal; it's more of a knee-jerk reaction to unexpected change than anything else. If you stick to your program and start showing measurable results, you might just be the one who leads your entire coffee klatch up off the sofa and into the gym.

The Mind-Body Connection

Dozens of scientific studies have proven over and over that our bodies and our minds are intricately bound to each other in ways we are only beginning to understand. No one even bothers to question the idea any more; it's accepted for the truth that it is.

But for years this was not so. We had no idea that our minds and our bodies were connected in any way other than a mechanical one. We knew our brain could tell our legs to move or our throat to swallow, but we didn't realize that it could essentially orchestrate a breakdown of physical systems that resulted in illness. And yet this is just what our brains do when subjected to unrelenting stress over a period of time—release hormones and chemicals that can trigger debilitating illness in our physical bodies by suppressing our immune systems.

Stress Kills

Cortisol, the hormone that flows throughout your body whenever you feel stressed, is essential for regulating numerous bodily functions including blood pressure and heartbeat. But when your body produces an oversupply of this powerful hormone in response to too many stress triggers, the results can be devastating to your health.

Fortune magazine estimated that stress and stress-related illnesses cost American businesses an average of $150 billion a year. Insurance companies claim that 70 to 90 percent of all medical claims by insured workers are for stress-related illnesses or injuries. They calculate that they could reduce benefits claims by up to 30 percent if people made some simple lifestyle changes to manage their stress.

Business executives are beginning to understand the serious implications of stress in the workplace. While some may scoff at the idea of an on-site masseuse or counselor, statistics prove that providing employees with outlets for their stress and giving them tools to better manage the stress that remains pays off in lower absenteeism and fewer medical claims.

Head First, Body Next

There's an important reason why experts recommend that you straighten out your thinking and attitude before you attempt any major changes in your life. If you do it backward and try to work on your body before you have shaken the cobwebs out of your head, your mind will have a tendency to sabotage whatever efforts you are making to change. That's because our bodies exist in a biological state known as *homeostasis* or balance. We naturally fight against anything that would tend to change that state of balance.

Wellness Words

Homeostasis is a relatively stable state of equilibrium or a tendency toward such a state between the different but interdependent elements or groups of elements of an organism, population, or group.

Homeostasis plays a vital role in keeping all our systems in balance, but it can work against us when we are trying to make changes, even if those changes are beneficial. Be aware of the role that homeostasis plays in keeping you stuck wherever you are, and remember that it takes a full three weeks to retrain your brain into thinking and behaving in a new way.

A Whole New World

When you straighten out your thought processes and replace self-destructive behaviors with healthy behaviors that enhance your wellness, you will find yourself in a whole new world. As your physical appearance and feelings of wellness continue to improve, your self-confidence will skyrocket. You may be surprised to find real joy as an everyday component of your life.

Once you have adjusted your attitude and are starting to see the results of incorporating healthier behaviors into your life, you'll find yourself with a little time on your hands. This is the time that you used to spend worrying and stressing over your health and lifestyle. At this point, it is natural to turn inward and start examining matters of the heart and soul, what some people call the spirit. It is now that you will ask yourself the really hard questions relating to your core beliefs: Am I happy with the choices I have made in my life? Am I at a point where I can make some different choices? Do I feel comfortable making these changes?

This transition can be particularly important for members of the baby boom generation. We were raised in relative luxury and taught to work and play hard. We rarely allowed time for introspection. Now, as we enter our 40s, 50s, and 60s, it is natural for us to start assessing our lives and trying to figure out if there are some changes we can make for the better. It's truly the boomers who are driving this current interest in wellness and whole-ness.

If you've got your head on straight and your body looking better than ever, you may ask yourself why it's even necessary to look inward. We've said from the beginning that this book is about the mind-body-spirit connection and seeking wellness in all three areas. True peace arises from balancing all three.

It is true that you can change your spirit without changing your mind or your body, but why would you want to? Do you really want to house your newfound joy and sense of purpose in a "cracked vessel"?

The most wonderful thing about true wellness is that it frees the spirit. Achieving wellness is like letting a bird out of a cage; it allows your spirit to soar without physical or mental limitation to the highest reaches of your potential. Wellness allows you to reach your true destiny.

The Least You Need to Know

- ◆ Wellness provides benefits that can positively affect almost every area of your life.
- ◆ Successful wellness programs start in your head.
- ◆ It takes 21 days of repeating the same behavior to break a bad habit or form a new and hopefully beneficial habit.
- ◆ It's natural for your friends to try to distract you from your wellness goals.
- ◆ The current focus on wellness is driven by the millions of baby boomers now entering their 40s, 50s, and 60s.

Part 2

The First Pillar—Nutrition—You Really Are What You Eat

Diet really is a four-letter word, because when some people hear the word *diet*, they run screaming in the opposite direction. So we're not going to use that word too frequently in this section, except to talk about the sort of fad diets that can be so detrimental to your health.

What we are recommending instead is to take a look at your overall nutritional plan to see if the way you are eating now truly supports optimal health. If, as we suspect, it does not, we have lots of tips and information to share—everything from an overview of nutrition to the latest recommendations for vitamin and mineral supplements to ways to reform if you're a sugarholic or junk food addict.

And no, eating right doesn't mean you are condemned to a lifetime of tofu burgers and bean sprouts. It just means making thoughtful choices and being sure to include a variety of fresh foods in your daily meal planning. And here's one final hint: Nutritious food is not only good for you, but actually tastes better than that junky stuff.

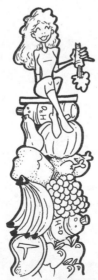

Chapter 5

The Importance of Proper Nutrition in Maintaining Wellness

In This Chapter

- ◆ It's just food, right?
- ◆ The building blocks of health
- ◆ How junk food makes you sick
- ◆ Eating your way to wellness

Tell us there's a person among you who hasn't at one point or another scarfed down an entire pint of Häagen-Dazs, box of Oreos, or bag of chips in one sitting. Tell us you can resist putting extra onions *and* cheese on top of your bowl of firehouse chili or stop at just one helping of turkey, stuffing, mashed potatoes, and pumpkin pie at Thanksgiving.

What's that we hear? Thundering silence? We thought so.

We're only human, and humans, like all other mammals, enjoy eating. It's our style of eating that gets us into trouble; we eat too much and tend to load up our plates with foods that don't have much bang for the buck. In other words, we eat foods that are high in calories but relatively low in nutritional value. Worse yet, many of the foods we favor are actually detrimental to our health because they contain such high levels of saturated fat, sugar, or sodium or too many chemicals and artificial additives that our bodies can't process.

There's no getting around it. What you do or don't eat is vitally important to your health. In fact, nutrition is so important we have made it our first pillar of wellness.

Why Does It Matter What I Eat?

You may be wondering why it even matters what you eat. What's the difference anyway? Food is food, right?

Wellness Words

The word *nourish* means "to maintain, sustain, or promote growth." So when we call food **nourishment,** we're not just talking about something we put in our mouths to satisfy our hunger. We're talking about something that sustains our very lives; we're talking about our fuel.

Actually, food is nutrition, or better yet, *nourishment,* not only for our bodies but also for our senses and our spirits. While we may not be able to tell much difference between the 13 grams of saturated fat we get from a 1-ounce bag of chips and the 14 grams of monounsaturated fat we get from 1 tablespoon of olive oil, our bodies sure can.

The olive oil contains oleic acid, an essential fatty acid that has been proven in numerous studies to lower the serum levels of LDL or "bad" cholesterol and raise the serum levels of HDL or "good" cholesterol. In addition, it contains:

- **Tocopherals.** Various forms of vitamin E in a balanced combination that is readily available to your body.
- **Polyphenals.** Antioxidants that help your body fight free radicals and which may help slow the aging process by inhibiting the cell- and DNA-damaging process of oxidation.
- **Squalene.** An important component in helping the body regulate its metabolism.
- **Triolein.** A bioactive lipid that helps your body easily absorb olive oil and all its nutrients.
- Plus many other minerals and nutrients that help maintain good health in amounts so minute they are identified only as "traces." However, your body needs and uses these traces on a daily basis to continue functioning optimally. It is these traces that are extremely difficult to replicate accurately in nutritional supplements, no matter how carefully they are formulated.

Here's how the chips stack up nutritionally. In addition to the saturated fat from the hydrogenated oils used to fry the things, the chips also contain:

◆ High levels of sodium (salt)
◆ High levels of simple carbohydrates that convert to sugar and cause a spike of insulin in your blood

Over time, hydrogenated oils and other saturated fats can lead to a buildup of arterial plaque, which can cause heart attacks. Excessive salt intake can contribute to the development of high blood pressure and kidney problems. Eating a lot of simple carbohydrates and sugars has been directly implicated in the development of adult-onset Type II diabetes. New studies suggest this sort of diet can also make people fat and more susceptible to a variety of cardiovascular diseases.

Still convinced it doesn't matter what you eat? Still want those chips?

CAUTION 911!

If you want to reduce your risk of a heart attack, stay away from eating large, high fat meals. A new study shows the excess fatty particles circulating in your blood after a high-fat meal may interfere with blood flow to the heart and trigger a heart attack. A recent study of 2,000 heart attack victims in Boston found their risk for suffering a heart attack increased by as much as 4 to 10 times in the 2 hours following a large, heavy, fatty meal. To safeguard your cardiovascular health, moderate fat intake at each meal and stop eating before you feel overstuffed.

But It Tastes So Good!

For some reason, we seem to believe anything that's good for you has to taste awful and everything delicious is automatically bad for you. Nothing could be farther from the truth. If you compare the taste of a chicken breast freshly sautéed with mushrooms and onions in a little bit of olive oil to the taste of a frozen "chicken breast" made out of heaven knows what parts, complete with cardboard veggies and a large helping of chemical preservatives and stabilizers, the one you cook yourself will win the taste test every time.

Scientists consider taste to be the most complex human sense; it's certainly the one they understand the least. The fact that our gustatory sensors, or taste buds, are hot-wired with our olfactory sensors, or noses, just makes things more complicated. The best meals are those that appeal to both our sense of taste and our sense of smell. In fact, odor comes first. If the aroma of a dish doesn't appeal to us, we probably will not put even one bite of the food into our mouths.

This aroma-taste connection is one reason why fragrant herbs like rosemary and mint are so popular in cooking and why vegetable seasonings like onion and garlic are staples in wildly diverse cultures. When food smells good, it tantalizes our appetites and makes us want to sit down and partake. When it smells bad, it triggers a primitive warning center in our brains that was originally meant to keep us from eating spoiled food. Too bad it doesn't work for junk food.

Biology and Habit Control Your Taste Destiny

Taste buds contain cells that allow us to detect and distinguish salty, sour, sweet, and bitter sensations. We tend to associate taste buds with our tongues, but the roof of our mouths and the insides of our cheeks also have taste buds, which make tasting truly a "whole mouth" experience.

How we experience taste is very much a function of the number and array of taste buds we have in our mouth, and that, in turn, is a function of genetics and heredity. That's why something that tastes wonderful to one person can literally turn another person's stomach; it's also why people in the same family tend to have similar food preferences.

Believe it or not, the average human tongue contains 184 taste buds per square centimeter, although some poor souls, known as nontasters, only have 96. Then there are other people, primarily women, known as "supertasters," who have as many as 425 taste buds per square centimeter on their tongues. Supertasters can easily find employment working in industries, where consistency of taste is vital to maintain a product's reputation.

There is a downside to being a supertaster though; since the number of pain receptors in the tongue is directly tied to the number of taste buds, supertasters are likely to experience hot or spicy foods as a painful experience. That explains why some people can chomp down jalapeños with abandon while the same relatively mild pepper might send a supertaster to the emergency room.

Despite the wide array of available spices, including jalapeños, we Americans have gotten used to the artificial taste of the chemicals commonly used as preservatives. We rely so heavily on packaged and prepared convenience foods that those foods with stale tastes or off odors or flavors pass right by us. As long as it comes in a little cellophane wrapper or box and can be nuked in a microwave and ready to eat in two minutes, we'll buy it and stick it in our mouths.

Through trial, error, and bitter experience, I have learned to rely upon my own devices when it comes to my care and feeding. My definition of something that tastes bad is any food that's been sitting in a carton on a grocer's shelf for a year or two—or even a week or two. When it comes to food, fresh tastes best. And remember, "good for you" doesn't have to equal "tastes like blown insulation." Get that idea out of your head right now.

Who Has Time to Cook?

Fresh is best, and that brings us around to the sticky subject of cooking. In today's mad, mad world, who has time to cook? The answer is, we all do, and if we care about our health, we all should. Yes, it takes some planning ahead, but the results are worth the effort. And no, you do not have to be Martha Stewart to prepare delicious, healthy meals very quickly and efficiently.

Let's face it. We all work way too many hours; many of us think of our kitchens only as that place where we store our expensive but rarely used set of matched gourmet cookware or that room we dash into every once in a while to microwave popcorn or brew a cup of instant coffee.

Would you be interested in taking on the responsibility of feeding yourself and your family if we told you that you could plan and prepare an entire week's worth of delicious, healthy meals in the equivalent of an hour or less per day? Is your health and satisfaction worth an investment of seven hours a week of your time?

We think it is, and we're going to tell you just how to do it in Chapter 9, "Planning Healthy Snacks and Meals."

Good Nutrition Makes Good Bodies

We all love our families and want to do the best we can for them. So think of cooking nutritious meals as a way of not only showing that love but also as a way to give your children (and yourself) everything needed to grow strong and stay healthy. The same philosophy should hold true even if you live alone; you deserve the best and most nutritious food well prepared. Even if you are not a cook, with a few simple tips you can easily prepare meals fit for royalty.

From the Medicine Chest

The skin covering our bodies is entirely renewed every 28 days. All our other organs and systems renew themselves regularly as well. Our bodies need high-quality building blocks to keep performing these miraculous feats of repair and renewal. It's not as if our cells can run down to the local Home Depot and pick up a quart of collagen or fibrinogen whenever they need it. Our bodies synthesize the building blocks they require from the foods we eat. When we eat unwisely we deny our bodies the nutrients they need to stay well and keep renewing themselves. Without adequate replacement materials on hand, we are more susceptible to systemic breakdown and disease. Injuries heal more slowly, and recovery from illness takes longer. By regularly choosing and eating poor-quality foods, we are actually hastening our own aging and degeneration process.

The simple truth is that good nutrition builds healthy bodies. To enhance wellness and discourage the onset of illness, we should select and eat a good variety of nutritious foods to supply our bodies with the building blocks they need to keep us in good repair.

Food Nourishes Us, Body and Soul

Why do we eat? Simply to satisfy our physical hunger? No. Another big reason we eat is for enjoyment—the pleasure of experiencing tantalizing aromas and flavors, the satisfaction of feeling full after a wonderful meal.

In addition, there's the social side of eating. Even if you occasionally eat alone, eating is meant to be a joyous experience, not this 90-mile-per-hour dash through a drive-thru we have reduced it to in the twenty-first century.

One of the biggest things standing between us and the enjoyment of a good meal is that we eat too darned fast. Americans tend to wolf down their food, barely stopping to breathe in between bites. This tendency to race through meals is probably one reason why our food manufacturers have gotten away with providing such lousy fare for so long—we don't bother to taste our food; we simply inhale it.

Europeans have a tendency to snicker at this particular American tribute. When I was a college student, I lived in Bologna, Italy, for almost a year. I took intensive Italian lessons for several weeks after I first arrived. After we achieved some proficiency in speaking, our instructor sat us around a large table and asked questions that we were expected to answer in Italian. This daily practice rapidly improved our language skills.

One day she asked us how long we were given to eat lunch in our native countries. The Italian students answered four or five hours, which was the length of their *intervallo* or lunch break. Lunch is a real production in Italy, the big meal of the day. I don't know how it is now, but in the mid-1970s, Italian fathers came home from work to eat the huge lunch that the Italian mothers had spent all morning preparing. Everyone ate until they were cross-eyed, then retired for a two-hour nap.

Scientists say that your brain needs up to 20 minutes to receive the "full" message from your stomach. If you eat slowly, taking the time to savor the taste of each bite and chew thoroughly before swallowing, you will give your brain enough time to receive the "full" signal. If you shovel in your food, barely pausing for air between bites, by the time your brain receives the "full" signal you will actually be overstuffed and feeling quiet uncomfortable. If you want to reduce your risk of heartburn, indigestion, and the other unpleasant side effects that

Health Notes

A new study by Nielsen NetRatings showed that office Internet use dips during lunch breaks in Europe when employees tend to leave the building for the extended, leisurely lunches that are typical there. But American office Internet use showed no corresponding dip, which means that some people skip lunch altogether so they can have more time to surf the Net.

can result from eating too much too fast, slow down and chew slowly. An added bonus is that by eating slowly you will greatly reduce the number of calories you take in without feeling hungry or deprived, which is a big help in weight management.

One of the biggest problems with eating too fast is that it greatly increases the odds of a choking incident. The so-called "café coronary" causes almost 2,000 deaths per year. According to the Center for Disease Control, choking on food accounts for almost 70 percent of all choking incidents. The most common culprits are hot dogs, nuts, vegetable and meat pieces, fruit, and hard candy. All the more reason to slow down and chew thoroughly.

Symptoms of choking include the following:

- Inability to talk
- Wheezing
- Forceful coughing
- Clutching the throat or chest as a sign of distress
- Loss of consciousness
- Cyanosis

If someone is choking, call 911 and administer the Heimlich Maneuver:

1. Lean the person forward slightly and stand behind him.
2. Make a fist with one hand.
3. Put your arms around the person and grasp your fist with your other hand near the top of the stomach, just below the center of the ribcage.
4. Make a quick, hard movement, inward and upward.

If this does not dislodge the food, try to clear the airway with your fingers and administer CPR until help arrives.

Don't you think it's crazy that we try to cram one of life's greatest pleasures into 15-minute boxes? Make a pledge to yourself that you are going to slow down and really enjoy your next meal. We think you will be pleasantly surprised with your results.

Prescription for Illness

Our bodies are designed to work a certain way and require specific nutrients to keep functioning correctly. If we continually deny our bodies the fuel they need, and instead substitute inferior-quality foods that "gunk up" our "engines," over time that engine is naturally going to develop problems.

There are certain things ubiquitous in the American diet that one would be hard-pressed to find in food in any other country. The primary culprits here are hydrogenated oils, the cheap emulsifiers that American food manufacturers have been using as food preservatives since the mid-1950s. Some studies suggest that as much as 90 percent of the packaged foods available in the typical American grocery store contain hydrogenated or partially hydrogenated oils as preservatives.

From the Medicine Chest

During the process of hydrogenation, hydrogen atoms are moved to the opposite side of the double bond of the fatty acid's molecular structure, creating what is now known as a "trans-fatty acid," *trans* meaning the atoms have been moved "across" the structure to a new location. This has the effect of making the oil solid or hard at room temperature. Although European countries limit by law the percentage of trans-fatty acids that a food may contain to 4 percent, there is no such protection in place for American consumers, who daily consume foods that contain as high as 50 percent trans-fatty acids. Denmark has banned hydrogenated oils in food preparation altogether.

For many years, hydrogenated oils were touted as healthy. Now we know better. A 14-year study of 85,000 nurses conducted by the Nutrition Department at the Harvard Medical School proved that the more trans-fatty acids people consume, the higher their rate of cardiovascular disease. A huge number of clinical studies performed at some of the most prestigious medical schools in the country implicates hydrogenated oils in the development of many diseases, including heart disease, cancer (particularly breast and colon cancer), diabetes, and several auto-immune disorders, among others.

The best nutritional advice we can give you to enhance wellness is to eliminate foods containing hydrogenated oils from your diet.

A Nation of Sugarholics

Fifteen years ago, the annual consumption of sugar in the United States was an average of 125 pounds per person. Today, it stands at a staggering 156 pounds per person per year, and that number is climbing annually.

Researchers have discovered that people who take in 15 percent or more of their daily calories in the form of sugar lose bone mass. The high sugar intake upsets their body chemistry and puts them in a negative calcium balance that causes their bodies to leech the calcium they need to function from their bones, contributing to osteoporosis. Excessive sugar consumption has also been linked to the development of adult-onset diabetes, hypoglycemia, hyperglycemia, and hyperinsulimia or resistance to insulin.

In addition, sugar causes cavities. Though the rate of cavities has been going down for school children in general, it is rising among children from lower-income families who don't have access to good dental care. Sadly, these are the same families who are likely to eat the poorest diets, a double whammy.

From the Medicine Chest

Like hydrogenated oils, sugars are hidden everywhere in packaged foods. It can be difficult to ferret them out because they are called by so many different names. Here are just a few:

- Fructose
- Sucrose
- Dextrose
- Glucose
- Lactose

Of course, you can always look for the total grams of sugar under the total carbohydrates listing on the label. Just remember this can be deceptive, because your body converts excess carbohydrates into sugar and then into fat for storage.

It is easier to manage your sugar intake when you prepare your own meals from fresh foods.

The High Cost of Convenience

It should come as no surprise to learn that America uses more convenience foods than any other country in the world. It would be wonderful to have such foods on hand for particularly busy evenings except for two things: They contain a lot of artificial preservatives that are damaging to health, and they are much more expensive than foods prepared from scratch. In one USDA survey, 3 pounds of store-bought potato salad cost $4.79, while the same amount of potato salad prepared at home from fresh potatoes cost just $1.59.

Experts advise that convenience foods generally cost anywhere from three to five times as much as the same amount of food prepared from scratch using fresh ingredients. An added bonus is that food prepared from scratch generally has a far superior taste and texture when compared to packaged foods that may have been prepared days or even weeks before.

911!

Beware that hydrogenated oil may go by another name on food labels. Mono-diglycerides are made from oils that have a high percentage of monounsaturated fats, but mono-diglycerides have been hydrogenated or chemically altered to remain solid at room temperature. Like other hydrogenated oil products, mono-diglycerides are used as preservatives.

The big barrier is time. We have ourselves convinced that it is faster and easier to plop six prebreaded chicken breasts onto a microwave plate and zap them than it is to take 15 minutes to sauté 6 fresh chicken breasts in a little olive oil and garlic. We don't think about the high cost of convenience—and we're not just talking about monetary costs, but also the cost to our overall health. With rare exception, prepackaged foods tend to be detrimental to health because of the number and nature of the chemical preservatives they contain. Convenient or not, those are risks none of us should be willing to take.

Do I Really Have to Give Up French Fries?

Every one of us has some less-than-healthful food we just adore and don't want to give up. It might be french fries, ice cream, chocolate, or chips. We love the taste, and we love the smell, the texture, the crunch, and the creaminess. Whatever it is, there is something about that food that comforts or excites us.

The key to these indulgent foods is moderation. Let's say your particular weakness is ice cream. If you ever tried to make yourself give it up entirely, your brain would implode. So instead of a bowl or cup of ice cream, dig out a nice big spoonful from the carton. Take it to your recliner, sit down, lean back, and enjoy. Make that spoon of ice cream last four or five minutes. At the end of that time, you will almost feel like you've had a four-scoop sundae. The key is to focus on enjoying the food and not on feeling bad because you are indulging one of your guilty pleasures.

So if french fries are your thing, by all means, dive in, but limit yourself to 10 or 15, and skip the "super-size" option.

Change Your Nutritional Habits to Change the Way You Feel

We hope by now you are convinced that you really do have the power to influence how well you feel by how well you eat. Even if you are the all-time champion junk food junkie, it's not too late to change your ways and start enhancing your wellness with better food choices.

It will take a bit of practice to actively increase your awareness of the importance of making wise food choices as you shop, but after a while, it will become second nature. You'll be able to pick up a carton or box and tell within a few seconds if it's something you want to add to your nutritional plan or not.

Make Eating Pleasurable

While you are busy changing what you eat, don't forget to change *how* you eat. There are lots of simple things you can do to make sure meals are pleasurable experiences. Once you start eating this way, you will never again want to go back to wolfing down food on the run.

If you take the time and make the effort to make your meals a special time, the benefits will be enormous. Even if your day is hectic, knowing that your meal time will be an oasis of calm, enjoyment, and relaxation can help pull you through.

For a wonderful, relaxing, and enjoyable meal, try the following:

- ◆ Use your best plates and glasses.
- ◆ Use cloth napkins.
- ◆ Put a fresh flower in a bud vase by each plate, or place a small centerpiece in the middle of the table.
- ◆ Dine by candlelight.
- ◆ Play soft music during the meal.
- ◆ Eat slowly and savor each bite.

To make a meal even more special, request the pleasure of the company of someone you truly care about.

Your Personal Dietitian

If you find all of this just too confusing to plow through, consider hiring a personal registered dietitian. The American Dietetic Association's website has a search feature that will help you find someone in your vicinity: www.eatright.org.

A registered dietitian can look at your current eating habits and help you develop a nutritional plan that is realistic for the amount of time, money, and effort you are willing to devote to the project.

The Least You Need to Know

- ◆ Every bite you put in your mouth has an effect on your body. Beneficial foods = good effects; junk foods = bad effects.
- ◆ Your body needs certain nutrients to be able to continually repair and renew itself. A well-balanced diet provides these nutrients; poor diets do not.
- ◆ Eating a poor diet over a long period of time will ultimately cause health problems.
- ◆ Eating wisely on a consistent basis will significantly enhance your feeling of wellness.

Chapter 6

Diet of the Week—an Overview of Current Diet Crazes

In This Chapter

- ◆ Psst! Wanna get rich? Write a diet book
- ◆ Follow the fads
- ◆ Dissecting the diets
- ◆ The importance of balance

Hardly a week goes by that the newspapers, magazines, and airwaves aren't full of news about the latest diet trends or fallout from a not-so-new fad diet that didn't end up being very effective. Ever hopeful, those of us who constantly battle our weight try first one diet and then another, but the outcome is almost always the same—failure.

The National Institute of Diabetes and Digestive and Kidney Diseases reports that only 5 percent of people who lose weight manage to keep it off for at least a year. Every one else gains it all back, usually with an additional 5 or 10 pounds for good measure.

We don't need a scientific study to convince us that it's difficult to lose weight and even harder to keep it off. But that knowledge doesn't keep us from our constant search for the Holy Grail of diet books, *the* one that's going to have all the answers available at just the flip of a page. So how do you tell which diet books aren't worth the paper they are printed on and which might actually contain useful advice? We'll give you some guidelines in this chapter.

Diets Books: A Booming Business

There was a time when one of the quickest ways to get rich in America was to write a best-selling diet book. If your book claimed to help people lose a lot of weight very quickly with little or no effort on their part, no exercise required, and they didn't have to give up chocolate, your success was practically guaranteed.

We seem to be a little wiser now; while this could change at any time, we've just been through a rather extended period with no diet book hovering near the top of the nonfiction best-seller charts.

If you looked back over the history of best-sellers within the past decade or so, you would see that's unusual. Generally, there is some sort of diet book sitting atop *The New York Times* or *Publishers Weekly* best-seller lists, along with some high-profile physician, dietitian, personal trainer, or Hollywood star flogging their particular formula for weight loss.

A recent *Publishers Weekly* symposium of top health editors produced some telling points—baby boomers, that 77 million strong wave of humanity, were the ones pushing the diet craze. Now that they're entering their 40s, 50s, and 60s, their health concerns encompass more than simple weight loss. Industry pundits now predict a boom in a new kind of book, one that addresses the total health needs of a person, including weight management. Predictions are that this type of book will do much better in the future than whatever fad diet happens to crop up. But that doesn't mean there aren't people out there ready to fall for the "All Peanut Butter Diet." I know. I tried it. It was delicious. It didn't work.

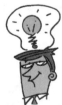

From the Medicine Chest

Search for the words *weight loss* at amazon.com and you'll get a list of 1,261 titles. We'll try almost any "miracle" pill, instant weight loss shake, slenderizing bar, herbal wrap, or bizarre machine anyone advertises. As long as they claim it will help us lose weight instantly without having to eat less or exercise more, we'll give it a go. According to the National Institute of Diabetes and Digestive and Kidney Diseases …

- More than half of U.S. adults are overweight, while nearly one-quarter are obese.
- Every year, approximately 50 million Americans go on a diet.

This makes us pretty fertile ground for someone hoping to launch a diet craze.

Of course, given Americans' problems with weight, there will always be a market here for diet pills, shakes, and bars and weight loss machines, books, and videotapes. But when it comes to fast or gimmicky weight loss claims, industry watchers think the buying public is less gullible these days. Part of the reason is the wide range of reliable information available on the Internet. People who have been scammed are likely to go into an online chat room and share their experiences or perhaps send e-mails to all their online friends. This sort of easy information exchange makes it harder for the scammers to perpetrate their frauds.

Another part of the reason is that people are tired of diets and dieting. We've tried them all: Atkins, Hollywood, Grapefruit, Cabbage Soup, SugarBusters!, the Zone, Somersizing, Weight Watchers, Jenny Craig, Nutrisystems, high protein, low protein, liquid protein, low fat, no fat—you name it. And guess what? We're fatter than ever. Most diets just don't work, not in the long run.

The diet industry loves Americans. We eat more than anyone else, we weigh more than anyone else, and we are loath to give up our daily ice cream and cookies (or chips and dip) just because they eventually might lead to a little old thing like a heart attack or cancer.

According to the Department of Nutrition at New York University, nearly one fourth of all new food products are developed with some health or nutritional goal in mind. But just because *they* say it's healthy doesn't mean that it's so. Several years ago, I was preparing a box of macaroni and cheese for my kids. I noticed the box was sporting a new sticker that claimed the product was "low fat." Huh? Macaroni and cheese prepared with butter and milk was low fat? I looked on the side of the box, and sure enough, they claimed each serving had just 4 grams of fat. Then I noticed another column that said each serving had 19 grams of fat "as prepared." That wasn't low fat at all. When I called the company to see what was going on, the customer service rep said the low-fat claim was only for the product as it came from the box, unprepared, with no butter or milk added.

Hmm, how many people do you know who eat their macaroni straight out of the box and raw? This company had been so eager to put a health food claim on its box that it didn't even stop to think through the implications of furnishing nutritional information for an uncooked product that no one eats uncooked.

Object lesson: Read the labels. No matter what fantastic claims a company prints on the front of the box, the truth is in the small print on the back of the box. In the end, it's up to you to decipher the claims and counterclaims made by food and supplement manufacturers. You'll be harder to fool if you're armed with solid information.

Just remember this one inescapable fact: It takes 3,500 calories to build 1 pound of human flesh. Every time you take in 3,500 calories more than what your body can metabolize and use for energy in any given day, you will gain a pound. Conversely, if you trim just 500 calories a day out of your food intake for a week, you will lose that pound. For example, cut back from 5 16-ounce sodas a day to 3 (save 200 calories), eat half a bagel instead of a whole bagel every morning (save 100 calories), and eat 1 big scoop of ice cream every night instead of 2 (save 225 calories), and you will save more than 500 calories a day. No deprivation, just moderation, and at the end of one short week, you'll weigh 1 pound less. We'll talk more about this technique in Chapter 9, "Planning Healthy Snacks and Meals."

The Current Crazes

Of all the diet crazes that have come and gone over the years, one of the most enduring is the high-protein diet. Early liquid protein versions of this diet were actually deadly. In the late 1970s, liquid protein was blamed for at least 60 deaths, but the deaths were not due just to the extreme caloric restrictions of the diet (just 400 calories a day!), but rather to the fact that the diet put a severe strain on the kidneys, causing them to excrete too much water from the body.

Wellness Words

Electrolytes are non-metallic electrical conductors that convey electrical signals through the movement of ions. They keep the heart beating, blood flowing, lungs breathing, blood oxygenated, and other body processes working. Any disruption in the body's precisely balanced electrolyte array can result in cardiac arrhythmias or even sudden cardiac arrest.

This systemic "flush" swept out essential minerals from the bloodstream, which then produced an *electrolyte*, or body chemical, imbalance. Severe electrolyte imbalances can produce heart arrhythmias and even sudden cardiac arrest, and this is what killed these liquid protein dieters. It didn't help that the "protein" in these diets was a very poor quality derived from cowhides and gelatin. But it seems we will all try anything at least once.

In recent months, I have seen these diets advertised:

- Eat all you want and lose 40 pounds!!!
- Say good-bye to fat *and* wrinkles!
- The Amazing Peanut Butter diet!
- Turn off your hunger and lose seven pounds a week!
- Eat to lose and drop all the weight you want!
- Super-fat weight loss! Lose seven pounds in three days!
- Melt away belly fat!
- The Water Cure! Drink away 40 pounds!

And my personal favorite, in a magazine dated December 2:

- Lose 20 pounds by Christmas!

This last one was supposedly accomplished by following the "cellulite-melting secrets" of The Rockettes.

Hmm, where do I begin? First of all, you can't "eat all you want" and lose any weight, much less 40 pounds. Second, diets that emphasize one food to the exclusion of others contribute to nutritional imbalances, which can be dangerous. Third, all rapid weight loss is due to water depletion, which can itself cause health problems because your body needs water to run properly. And yes, while we do *need* water, you cannot drink away weight unless your increased water intake is accompanied by decreased caloric intake. Fourth, when you lose weight, you lose it from all over your body. There are no "special foods" that burn fat only from your belly or your thighs. Finally, cellulite doesn't melt. Period.

CAUTION

911!

> Any diet that promises rapid weight loss is actually depending on rapid water loss to be effective. Although you may see a difference on the scale, these diets won't make a dent in your stored fat and can lead to dangerous electrolyte imbalances. Experts say we can safely lose up to two pounds a week. Any more than that may be dangerous and misleading, because it's probably not fat you're losing, but water, along with many essential trace minerals your body needs to maintain essential functions.

You know the old adage, "If it sounds too good to be true, it probably is"? Well, nowhere is this saying more relevant than in the world of fad diets. Here are a few sound principles to help you pick your way through the minefield of diet crazes:

◆ Eat a balanced diet. In other words, eat a variety of foods from a variety of sources. Any diet that completely eliminates one category of foods or another is not healthy and will be almost impossible to keep up over time.

◆ Successful diets help people change their eating patterns from unhealthy, fat-producing habits to healthy, weight-loss, then healthy, weight-maintenance habits.

◆ Remember that eating is meant to be a pleasurable, enjoyable experience. Fad diets reduce eating to a set of inflexible rules, and that's no fun.

◆ A diet is nothing more than a way of eating. Good diets provide reasonable, enjoyable guidelines that are easy to follow for life; fad diets require difficult, sometimes bizarre food rituals that are virtually impossible to stick with for more than a few days or weeks at best.

Diet of the Week

It seems like there is some new wonder diet circulating around the water-cooler crowd or suburban coffee-klatches every week. Food-combining, Brussels Sprouts diet, diets tied to your blood type or your body type, diets that rely on mental control or divine intervention—you name it, somebody somewhere has already thought of it and written a book about it. Dieting is a huge business in this country, and the bigger we get, the bigger the diet industry gets.

> **Health Notes** _____
>
> According to the U.S. Department of Commerce, diet industry revenues have grown from an estimated $100 million annually in the 1950s to an estimated $50 billion in the 1990s. Prospects for the future of the diet industry are even brighter. The American Obesity Association reports that the prevalence of obesity in America has increased by more than 50 percent in the last 40 years. That's a lot of potential customers.

The Good, the Bad, and the Dangerous

Most health-care practitioners are aware that obesity and obesity-related illnesses account for almost 300,000 unnecessary, premature deaths in this country every year. Not as well known is the fact that another several hundred people also lose their lives each year as a result of following an ill-advised fad diet or taking diet pills, herbal weight loss teas, or some other "new and improved" but still potentially deadly weight loss gimmick.

We don't even like the word *diet*, we prefer *nutritional plan*. Still, if you must diet, there are some plans that definitely stand out from the rest. Despite all the hoopla that might lead you to think otherwise, there are basically five types of diet plans:

- High protein, high fat, low carb—Atkins, Protein Power
- High protein, moderate carb—the Scan Diet, the Zone, SugarBusters!
- High protein, moderate to high fat, moderate to high carb—the Carbohydrate Addict's Diet
- Very low fat—the Ornish program, Pritikin Diet
- High carb, moderate fat—Weight Watchers, Jenny Craig

Although people come up with different combinations all the time, these profiles fit just about every currently popular diet. Now let's examine them and determine the pros and cons of each.

The Good

Let's start with the good. No less an authority than the U.S. Department of Agriculture (USDA) recently came out and declared that a high-carb, moderate-protein, moderate-fat plan (like Weight Watchers) was the healthiest diet out there, and the one most likely to produce successful, sustainable results. Dieters who follow this plan get about 55 percent of their calories from complex carbohydrates, 25 percent from fat, and about 15 to 20 percent from protein.

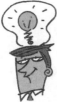

From the Medicine Chest

One good way to track your food intake is to keep a simple food journal. Buy a plain notebook, write the day's date at the top of each page, and simply write down everything you eat and drink over the course of the day. In addition, note how you are feeling throughout the day—if you develop a headache, indigestion, get fatigued—write all of that down.

Recording your food intake and how you feel takes only a few minutes over the course of the day and could reward you with significant information about your own food sensitivities and health.

Of course, the USDA may love this diet because it promotes approximately the same proportions of food intake that its own Food Pyramid recommends. Setting aside the ring of government authority for a few moments, it's important to know there has been recent controversy over whether or not the Pyramid is self-serving. The USDA's job, say some critics, is to promote the dairy, beef, and agricultural industries of our nation, so naturally their Pyramid will focus heavily on those products.

Nonetheless, according to government statistics, people who follow the USDA Food Pyramid *and* engage in regular exercise do quite well in managing their weight and avoiding serious illness.

Take the same diet and remove exercise from the equation, and you will suddenly find yourself with an increased risk of heart disease, because high carbohydrate intake without regular exercise raises serum triglyceride levels and promotes irregularities in blood sugar.

No one denies that both the Pritikin and Ornish diet programs can actually reverse heart disease; that's been proven clinically. The problem is that it requires extraordinary self-discipline to adhere to either of these programs because they are so restrictive. However, if you find yourself in a life-threatening situation because of cardiovascular disease, following either the Pritikin or Ornish plan could add years to your life.

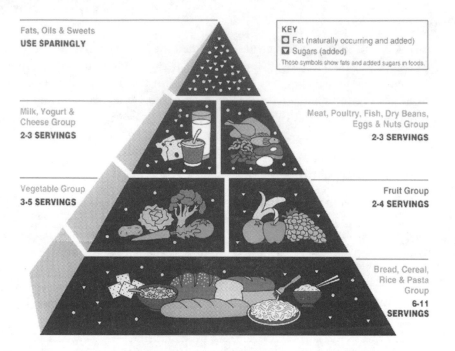

The U.S. Department of Agriculture recommends a balance of foods that is very similar to that recommended by Weight Watchers.

(Courtesy of USDA)

The Bad

Now let's take a look at the bad. Any diet that requires you to forever give up one category of food is generally a bad diet because you will not be able to stay on it for very long. Of course there are dietary restrictions that are medically based, such as the requirement that diabetics stay away from foods containing excessive amounts of sugar, like baked goods, sodas, or candy. But for anything other than a medical reason, restrictive diets are generally not a good idea.

When we are talking about natural foods, there is really no such thing as a "bad" food. And by natural, we don't mean something you bought from the health food store. We mean food in its original unadulterated state, just as it came from the ground or the sea or the vine or the tree or from the cow or the chicken. Any diet that characterizes any food or food group as "bad" is in fact, bad itself. Be wary if you run across a food plan that says, "strawberries are poisonous to humans" or "milk causes disease." Although there are some people who suffer from allergies that make milk or strawberries a forbidden food, no food has been proven to be "bad" for the general population.

Furthermore, diets like SugarBusters! (Ballantine Books, 1998) and the Scan Diet (GNC Stores) are difficult to stay on, because they eliminate too many categories of foods that people like. Most diets consider carrots to be a healthy addition. SugarBusters! makes them a forbidden food because they have a high *glycemic index*. Glycemic index was the buzzword in diet circles for a couple of years. All foods with a high glycemic index were forbidden. Then researchers discovered that determining a food's glycemic index in a test tube had nothing to do with the way a human body would process and utilize that food. The lab tests didn't take into account things like dietary fiber, which greatly affects the way a body metabolizes a particular food. The Scan Diet requires you to drink five shakes a day. No matter how much you like shakes, eventually you long for something else. At almost $3 per shake packet, this is one of the most expensive diets around.

Wellness Words

The **glycemic index** is a measure of how rapidly a food is digested and how quickly its sugar content gets into the bloodstream. Foods with a high glycemic index are digested rapidly, and their sugar content floods the bloodstream quickly. Foods with a lower glycemic index take longer to digest and to release their sugar content into the blood.

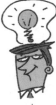

From the Medicine Chest

If you're looking for an easy way to compare the pros and cons of various diets, the U.S. Department of Agriculture has posted an executive summary of their recent overview of the subject at www.usda.gov/news/releases/2001/01/whitepaperexe.htm. Their conclusion is that we don't know nearly enough about the available dietary programs, but based upon what evidence we do have, the USDA concluded that while it is possible to lose a few pounds on almost any diet, the results achieved from most programs are not sustainable.

One of the craziest current diets is the Carbohydrate Addict's Diet (New American Library, 1999). It recommends a breakfast and lunch of almost pure protein and fat, followed by a "reward meal" that can be anything you like, as many calories as you like, and as much carbohydrate and sugar as you like, as long as you complete the meal within one hour. We've seen people gain a lot of weight on this diet because they were using the unrestricted "reward meal" as an excuse to pig out. If you're eating 2,000 or 3,000 calories at one meal you're not going to lose weight ever, no matter how much you starve yourself at breakfast and lunch.

There's a new prescription drug called Xenical, which is supposed to block absorption of up to 30 percent of the fat content in the food you eat. Experts decry this for two reasons. First, Xenical and other similar drugs do not teach you healthy eating habits, but instead allow you to rely on a chemical purgative to get rid of any excess fat you consume. Second, Xenical produces frequent, loose, and occasionally even uncontrollable bowel movements, often accompanied by painful cramps and bloating.

Chitosan is similar to Xenical in that it blocks absorption of some fat in the large bowel and has similar though less dramatic side effects and causes dependence just as Xenical does.

The Dangerous

Unfortunately, the people who come up with the various diet programs and weight loss supplements rarely have your health and safety as their primary consideration. Every year, well-meaning but misguided people lose their lives to one diet fad or another. The latest tragedy involved a drug combination popularly known as fen-phen. Experts believe as many as a thousand people lost their lives to this drug combination, and thousands more suffered permanent health consequences.

> **CAUTION**
>
> **911!**
>
> If you used the fen-phen drug combination to lose weight, you may be at risk for significant health problems. According to the Mayo Clinic, as many as 30 percent of the people who took fen-phen may have damage to their heart valves or pulmonary arteries. The drugs' manufacturer, American Home Products, has established a $4 billion fund to settle claims. If you took this drug, contact an attorney or e-mail info@FenPhenSettlements.com to discover if you should have an echocardiogram and to get additional information.

It's interesting to note that the combination of Fenfluramine (Pondamin), an appetite suppressant, and Phentermine (Fastin, Adipex, Zantryl), a mild stimulant, was never actually approved by the FDA for use as a diet drug, but rather was something doctors started prescribing after anecdotal evidence concerning its appetite suppressive effects became widespread. This is known as an "off-label" prescription because the drug is being prescribed for something that was not described in its original patent application.

You may be thinking to yourself, well, I took fen-phen and nothing bad happened to me, and that may well be true. But if you took it for two months or more, there's a chance the popular combination of drugs caused heart valve damage or primary pulmonary hypertension (PPH). The first symptoms may not show up for years, and by the time they do, the dizziness, fatigue, breathlessness, chest pain, and swelling are often attributed to the patient's weight problem rather than the underlying damage caused by the drug combination. More than 50,000 lawsuits filed by patients who suffered cardiopulmonary damage as a result of taking fen-phen have already been settled, and thousands more are pending.

Ephedrine is another popular diet supplement ingredient that has come under recent fire. The FDA says it caused nine deaths in 2001, and they recently moved to restrict the amount of ephedrine that can be included in supplements. Ephedrine was the active ingredient in a number of so-called "herbal fen-phen" preparations that were marketed in health food stores at the same time fen-phen was being prescribed by thousands of doctors. It can cause cardiac arrhythmias and sudden cardiac arrest.

And now we come to the famous Atkins Diet (*The Atkins Diet Revolution: Refined and Improved*, Avon, 2001). Dr. Atkins predated even the liquid protein craze. His 1972 book, *The Atkins Diet Revolution*, advocated a high protein intake accompanied by a near-total shunning of carbohydrates of any sort. It became popular because such a diet *does* cause rapid weight loss, but you aren't exactly losing fat. Would such a diet seem so appealing to you if we explained that the way you lose weight on such a diet is by actually digesting your own muscles? Sounds pretty disgusting, but it's worse than that. By decreasing your lean muscle mass, the Atkins Diet actually sets you up for a huge weight gain when you finally get tired of the meat for breakfast, meat for lunch, meat for dinner, and meat for dessert routine.

Here's how it works: The Atkins Diet and most other high-protein, low- or no-carbohydrate diets are ketogenic. The lower carbohydrate intake is generally offset by a higher intake of fat, which in turn causes *ketosis*—our bodies manufactures ketones from fat in a desperate effort to fuel activity and prevent further breakdown of lean muscle tissue. Uric acid builds up in the blood as it competes with ketones for excretion through the kidneys, which can cause gout and even kidney failure. Severely restricted carbohydrate intake rapidly depletes glycogen stores in the liver and muscles, producing a huge water loss. It is this water loss combined with the breakdown of muscle tissue that causes the initial rapid weight loss associated with high-protein diets. But the bad news is that this sort of eating plan leaves the body's fat deposits virtually untouched.

 Wellness Words _____

Severe restriction of carbohydrate intake forces your body to go into a state of **ketosis,** in which it breaks down fat to produce energy, a very inefficient way of fueling the body. In ketosis, the body gets energy from ketones, minute carbon fragments or fuel the body has created from the breakdown of fat, something it does only in a last-ditch effort to preserve lean muscle mass. The body regards ketosis as an emergency state, when its normal pattern of creating fuel from glucose has been interrupted.

The other bad news is that high-protein diets are lacking many vital nutrients, so dieters are required to swallow dozens of pills every day just to stay healthy. Finally, these diets have been associated with nausea, weakness, electrolyte imbalances, constipation, severe dehydration, insomnia, calcium depletion (which can result in kidney stones), and other potentially serious kidney problems. Are a few pounds off the scale worth any of these risks?

We don't think so.

Maintaining Balance

It can be difficult to figure out the optimum balance between your protein and carbohydrate intake. A nutritional plan that works well for one person may not work quite as well for another, because we all have slightly different individual needs. This is where a food journal can come in handy. If you decide to follow a plan like the Zone, which recommends you get 40 percent of your calories from carbs, 30 percent from protein, and 30 percent from fat, you may not really be able to determine how effective the plan is unless you keep a food journal. You may find it difficult to hold your carb intake to 40 percent and discover that a simple bump-up to a 50 percent carb intake serves your personal needs better.

Diets are classified according to the percentages of each type of nutrient they allow:

Type of Diet	Fat	Carbohydrate	Protein
Low fat	Less than 10 to 19 percent	More than 65 percent	10 to 20 percent
Moderate fat	20 to 30 percent	55 to 60 percent	15 to 20 percent
High fat	55 to 65 percent	Less than 20 percent	25 to 30 percent

Source: U.S. Department of Agriculture

The Atkins Diet is considered a high-fat diet, while Pritikin is low-fat. Most diet plans recommend nutrient percentages in the moderate-fat range.

The safest diets are ones that recommend a balance of nutrients. Any time a diet recommends an extreme imbalance or suggests you confine your diet to just one type of food, your warning flags should go up.

Don't Go Overboard

When considering which diet or nutritional plan works for you, just remember to keep it all in perspective and that eating should be an enjoyable activity. When you have to worry about every single bite you put in your mouth, you can't enjoy a meal. And that's exactly the problem with so many of these complex diets that require particular food combinations, or that only allow you to eat certain foods at certain times of the day.

In deciding which carbohydrates to include in your nutritional plan, remember that quality counts. Whole grains and cereals and fresh fruits and vegetables all contain high-quality carbohydrates along with a natural supply of vitamins, minerals, and fiber. Low-quality carbs don't have much of the good stuff but do contain plenty of health-destroying gunk like hydrogenated oils, chemical preservatives, simple sugars, and artificial colorants. Which would you rather have? (We already know which your body desires.)

Yes, including high-quality carbs in your diet does require a bit more planning than grabbing a Twinkie and a cup of java off the coffee cart, but these days, coffee carts are just as likely to offer a bowl of fresh fruit as a tray of donuts or cookies. Make it a habit to reach for the apple instead of the apple muffin, and your body will thank you.

The Least You Need to Know

- The diet industry has a vested interest in keeping Americans fat.
- Just because a doctor puts his name on a diet doesn't mean it's healthy or safe.
- The best diets recommend a balance of nutrients chosen from among all the food groups.
- You should avoid any diet that characterizes any one of the food groups as "bad."

Chapter 7

Protein, Fats, and Carbs— What's the Optimum Balance?

In This Chapter

- ◆ Balancing food intake
- ◆ Proteins—high or low—which way to go?
- ◆ Good fat vs. bad fat
- ◆ The complexities of carbs

When we eat, we rarely stop to think about what we are putting in our mouths. As long as it looks reasonably appealing, smells okay, and doesn't taste too bad, we'll eat it. In the hectic pace of today's world, we are especially prone to eat things that require little or no preparation time. English translation: fast food.

But did you ever stop to think *why* we eat? Sure, it's to keep us from wasting away, but what we mean is, do you know what food does for your body? Are you aware that proteins, fats, and carbs each play specific and highly individualized roles in the running of your body? That's why a deficiency of any one can have a serious impact on your wellness.

In this chapter, we'll introduce you to the world of proteins, fats, and carbs and explain why defining and maintaining an optimum balance of these nutrients is so vitally important to your health.

Good Nutrition Is a Balancing Act

Figuring out the proper balance in your intake of proteins, fats, and carbs can be a daunting task. There is lots of conflicting advice out there about how to apportion your daily caloric intake among the three. Even nutritional experts cannot seem to reach a consensus on the subject.

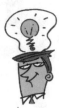

From the Medicine Chest

The human body requires a constant supply of nutrients to generate the energy it requires to keep going, to maintain and repair itself, and to support growth. When we are running low on one nutrient or another, hunger signals the body's need for more fuel.

Proteins, fats, and carbs each play different but equally important roles in the running, maintenance, and repair of the human body. Here's a quick guide to their jobs:

- **Protein.** Protein is your body's primary building block, an essential part of the structure of your skin, bones, and muscles. Proteins are used to renew and repair the body and to help synthesize the body's vital chemical messengers, including hormones and enzymes. They also play a crucial role in almost all your body's processes, including the transmission of nerve impulses and muscle movement.

- **Fats.** Far from being "bad," fats are so essential that life cannot exist without them. They are a vital component of our cells, the thing that allows cell walls to be permeable. That's important because permeability gives our bodies a way to hold water and nutrients within our cells while filtering out toxic wastes. Fats can also be burned to provide energy.

- **Carbohydrates.** Carbohydrates are the body's preferred fuel. They provide most of the energy required to run our bodies through a complex series of chemical reactions that start the moment we put a bite of carbohydrate-rich food into our mouths. Carbs are converted into a simple sugar called glucose that is carried to every cell in the body and used for energy.

Some argue that our diets provide two to three times the amount of protein humans actually need; others say there's no such thing as too much protein, and the typical American diet doesn't provide nearly enough. Some swear that a diet heavy in complex carbs is the way to go, while others believe such a diet is a recipe for disaster.

The U.S. Department of Agriculture (USDA) recommends as the optimum balance a moderate-fat, high–complex carbohydrate diet similar in composition to Weight Watchers and their own Food Pyramid. Their experts maintain this is the healthiest way to eat and also the type of program that allows people to take weight off and keep it off because it promotes healthy eating habits that can be sustained over the course of a lifetime.

The following table compares the USDA Food Pyramid to high-fat, high-protein, low-carb plans like Atkins and also to extremely low-fat plans like those promoted by Dr. Dean Ornish.

Type of Diet	Fat % of Calories	Carbohydrate % of Calories	Protein % of Calories
High fat, low carb (Atkins, etc.)	55 to 60	Less than 20	20 to 30
Moderate fat, high carb (Weight Watchers, USDA Food Pyramid)	20 to 30	55 to 60	15 to 20
Low fat or very low fat (Pritikin, Ornish)	10 to 19	More than 65	10 to 20

Source: USDA

The USDA also looked at how the typical American diet stacks up against the recommended balance of nutrients.

Type of Diet	Total Calories	% Fat	% Carbohydrate	% Protein
Typical American	2,200	35	50	15
High fat, low carb	1,414	60	10	30
Moderate fat, high carb	1,450	25	60	15
Low fat	1,450	10 to 15	65 to 75	15 to 20

Source: USDA

It's easy to see that the average American diet provides a higher number of daily calories that what we really need. It also contains a higher than recommended percentage of fat. The percentage of fat in the high-protein, high-fat, low-carb diets is almost off the map at 60 percent. The carbohydrate intake is so low that dieters who stay on the plan a long time may develop vitamin deficiencies because they are eating almost no fruits, vegetables, or grain products like bread or cereal.

Extreme Diets Have High Failure Rates

One of the main reasons people cannot stay on fad diets for long is that the dietary recommendations most of them provide are too complicated to follow. Over the long haul, it is difficult to maintain extreme imbalances in your eating patterns because people simply get tired of eating according to such rigid rules. They also rebel against the banning of many of their favorite foods. Sooner or later, the longing for familiar and comforting meals and snacks becomes overwhelming. If old eating habits have not been replaced by new, healthy, sustainable patterns of eating, going back to the old ways is just about inevitable. That's why the diet failure rate in this country is 95 percent.

Remember what we said back in Chapter 5, "The Importance of Proper Nutrition in Maintaining Wellness"—moderation, not deprivation. Let that be your mantra as you start to develop healthier eating habits. If you love chocolate, don't try to cut it out completely or you'll end up feeling so deprived that you'll eat it for breakfast, lunch, and dinner, and all the small meals in between. One lovely square savored slowly over the course of 10 minutes or so should be enough to satisfy your sweet tooth. And guess what? That square has about 80 calories and 1 gram of fat, numbers small enough to fit the treat into almost any nutritional plan.

> **CAUTION**
>
> **911!**
>
> If you never can seem to stick with a diet, don't blame yourself. According to the National Institute of Diabetes, Digestive and Kidney Diseases, for every 100 people who go on a diet, only 5 achieve any lasting success. That's because most diets require us to follow complicated and unfamiliar eating habits that are impossible to sustain over a lifetime.

Different Oats for Different Folks

So what's a poor, harried, time-constrained person to do? With so much confusing information out there, how can you decide what to eat and how to balance your diet?

Trial and error. Yes, we said "trial and error." You are the only one who knows what your stomach feels like after a particular meal. In Chapter 6, "Diet of the Week—an Overview of Current Diet Crazes," we suggested you keep a food journal to record your intake. You don't have to do it for the rest of your life, but just until you get a sense of what foods make you feel good and what foods give you problems.

Why can't you simply follow a plan from one of the hundreds of diet books out there and let it go at that? Because you are an individual, unique, and what works for other people might not work for you.

For example, let's take two 40-year-old women, both 5-foot-5, both 145 pounds. Betty whips up a protein shake with a piece of fresh fruit for breakfast every morning, while Thelma pours a bowl of whole-grain cereal topped with skim milk and a sliced banana.

Both options represent a healthy choice for breakfast, so why choose one over the other? Would it surprise you to learn that whole-grain cereals give Betty unbearable gas and that when Thelma tried protein shakes she developed a kidney stone? Each of these women has learned, through trial and error, what sort of food works best for her. Does that mean that whole-grain cereals and protein shakes are bad? No, simply that they may cause problems for certain individuals.

We may all be human, but we evolved from different tribes scattered all over the face of the earth. We originated from diverse climates with unique food supplies. As a result, our individual nutritional needs are slightly different. Books may give us the basics, a starting point to lay the foundation of a health-building nutritional plan, but it's up to each one of us to discover what our particular body needs to thrive.

There's an old adage that says "One man's meat is another man's poison." It is the literal truth. Some people can down bowl after bowl of chili with no apparent effect, while one spoonful would be enough to send another person into acute gastrointestinal distress. By keeping a food journal, you will soon know which foods are your "poisons," and learn to stay away from them. Something as simple as making an accurate observation of your food intake and correlating that intake with any resulting symptoms may be enough to permanently cure your recurrent heartburn, indigestion, or headaches.

Don't be afraid to chart your own nutritional course. In the end, you are the one person who is best qualified to determine what works for your body. Just don't try to convince us your body is calling out for three banana splits per day. We won't believe you, and you shouldn't believe you, either.

Stay the Course

As you start your journey to wellness, one of the most important things you can do is to figure out what foods your body needs and which you would do better to eliminate or eat only on occasion. Yes, this part is a bit tricky, but be faithful about keeping your food journal, and we promise that within two weeks, you will start to see patterns emerging that will give you invaluable information about your nutritional needs that you could not get any other way.

No matter how much you love a particular food, we would be willing to bet that if you have clear proof in your hands that that food causes you distress, you will soon lose your desire to eat it. Most of our problems with making poor food choices stem from the fact that we see no clear link between those choices and the way that eating them makes us feel. Keeping a food diary takes away our excuses. When the evidence is written in our own hands and gathered from our own acutely observed experiences, the information becomes much more powerful and difficult to ignore.

Protein—How Much Do We Really Need?

Muscles are built from protein. We must consume enough protein every day to keep our muscles healthy, in good repair, and capable of performing our normal daily tasks. The USDA says the ideal amount of protein for a healthy adult is 0.8 grams of protein per kilogram of body weight per day. Using this formula, a 175-pound man requires 64 grams of protein a day to maintain good health, while a 130-pound woman would need approximately 47 grams.

Children, pregnant and nursing women, elderly people, athletes, and anyone undergoing a stressful event like surgery or fighting a chronic disease like cancer needs more protein—up to 1 gram per kilogram of body weight per day.

There are fights raging in almost every corner of the nutrition world, but the fight over protein consumption is one of the fiercest. Since Dr. Atkins published his first high-protein, low- to no-carb diet book in 1972, the high-protein movement has steadily gathered steam. Experts say the diet's popularity stems from two things: It does cause a rapid early loss of weight (mostly water weight) due to the fact that it puts dieters into a state of ketosis by depriving their bodies of the preferred fuel source, glucose. When people almost entirely eliminate carbohydrates from their diets, the body has no choice but to start making ketones from fat to produce energy and to protect its lean muscle mass.

High Protein Can Equal High Fat

The other thing that makes the diet popular, especially with the meat-lovers crowd, is that foods we tend to think of as "forbidden" on other diets are encouraged on the Atkins Diet. Atkins dieters can have all the steak, bacon, turkey, pork, eggs, butter, cheese, or any other kind of protein they want because proteins do not trigger an insulin release into the bloodstream. Of course, as experts are quick to point out, eating all that protein comes at a price; because Atkins dieters eat so many saturated fats, the diet usually ends up raising their cholesterol levels. The rapid elimination of water through the urine caused by ketosis can lead to dehydration, which, in turn, can lead to the formation of kidney stones. In addition, when they finally tire of the all protein, all the time routine and start adding carbs back into their diets, they are likely to experience a very rapid regaining of the weight they lost because they haven't learned a healthy, balanced way to eat.

Hold the Mayo, and Give Me Your Strawberries

I once sat by an Atkins dieter at a business luncheon. She ordered a turkey sandwich on a bun, then asked for extra mayo and a bowl of strawberries with whipped cream for dessert. As I watched in horrified fascination, she took her sandwich apart, licked all the mayo off the bun, then discarded it along with the lettuce, tomatoes, and onions. She gobbled down the turkey and ate all the extra mayo from the little condiment cup with a spoon. Spying a few microscopic portions of mayo that had escaped her questing spoon, she ran her finger around the inside of the cup like a windshield washer, then noisily sucked the finger clean. Finally, and with great relish, acting as if she was the proud possessor of a "Get Out of Jail Free" card, she lapped down all the fake, chemical and preservative-laden "whipped cream" from the bowl of strawberries.

Leaving aside for the moment the question of manners, what was this woman really doing? She had somehow interpreted the Atkins mantra to mean that she could eat protein and fat with abandon as long as she eschewed carbs. No matter what anyone may tell you, calories do count. If you take in more of them in a day than your body can use, you will gain weight no matter what mysterious, magical combination of foods you eat.

As I watched with longing, the woman threw away the fragrant, gorgeous, red-to-the-rind strawberries because, as she told me in a conspiratorial whisper, they were carbs and, therefore, "evil."

We can't leave well enough alone. We refine food; add chemical stabilizers, taste enhancers, artificial dyes, flavorings, and preservatives; and beat just about every ounce of life out of it. But in their natural state the vast majority of fruits, vegetables, meats, poultry, fish, grains, and dairy products serve to enhance health, not damage it.

What Proteins Do

Unlike fats that can be stored in fat cells, or carbs that are broken down and stored as glucose or glycogen in the muscles and liver, the body has no place to store protein. We must take in an adequate amount of protein every single day or our bodies will start to break down. Of the 22 essential amino acids that combine to form proteins, 9 cannot be synthesized in the body; our diets must provide them. If they do not, we become protein deficient, a condition that produces a variety of unpleasant and even potentially deadly symptoms.

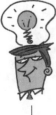

From the Medicine Chest

There are nine essential amino acids that our bodies cannot make: histidine, isoleucine, leucine, lysine, methionine, phenylalanine, threonine, tryptophan, and valine. These amino acids are used to create everything from collagen to bone, muscle, hair, and even our fingernails. All of our organs are in a constant state of repair and renewal. Protein plays the biggest role of all the nutrients in this ongoing rejuvenation process.

Symptoms of Protein Deficiency

There are very few of us who have trouble getting enough protein, although it can sometimes be a problem for vegetarians who do not closely monitor their diets. People who have inhibited appetites due to chronic illnesses or the side effects of a drug can also have trouble getting enough protein.

The symptoms of protein deficiency are varied and affect almost every system in the body. We'll list them from the mild to the serious:

- Brittle hair that falls out easily
- Brittle, ridged nails that break easily
- Flaky skin
- Slow healing of wounds
- Cold intolerance
- Diarrhea or constipation
- Muscle cramps
- Nausea
- Headaches
- Unexplained abdominal pain
- Swelling
- Muscle weakness and atrophy
- Weakness, fainting, and persistent fatigue
- Gallstones
- Gouty arthritis
- Elevated levels of uric acid in the blood
- Low blood pressure
- Increase in serum cholesterol levels
- Cardiac arrhythmias and other heart abnormalities

In addition, protein deficient diets can produce a host of mental symptoms including apathy, depression, irritability, moodiness, and a decrease in alertness, comprehension, and ability to concentrate.

Symptoms of Too Much Protein

Too much protein doesn't create quite the impressive list of symptoms that too little protein does, but the problems associated with excessive intake of protein can be quite serious. They include the following:

◆ Dehydration associated with ketosis

◆ Kidney stones

◆ Osteoporosis

We all go off the wagon occasionally. Last week I was invited to the opening of a local steakhouse. By the time I got through sampling the grilled chicken breast, mesquite-smoked sirloin, and succulent lobster tail, you can bet I had probably fulfilled my protein requirements for a week. The point is I rarely eat like that. I was right back on my recommended protein intake the next day and suffered no ill effects other than the apparent malfunction of my bathroom scale the next morning, which claimed I had gained three pounds. Hmm, must have been the cheesecake.

As long as you stick within 10 percent of your own recommended daily intake of protein on a fairly consistent basis, you should never have any trouble with the symptoms of too much or too little protein. Just remember to balance your diet with a varied intake of high-quality fats and complex carbohydrates as well.

Most Wanted: Healthy Fats

Over the past decade or so, dietary fats have gotten a bad rap in our culture. As a result, people have tried diligently to decrease their fat intake. Practically overnight, an entire new industry blossomed to produce an unending variety of "low-fat" or "fat-free" products to appeal to consumers' desire to decrease their fat intake. The problem is that removing the fat from food removes much of its taste appeal, so food manufacturers compensate by adding lots of sugar and chemical taste enhancers. The end result? After more than a decade of watching our fat intake, we Americans weigh more than ever and are unhealthier than ever. So whatever we've been doing hasn't worked; in fact, religiously following a low-fat or no-fat regimen over a period of time can produce some nasty health consequences.

Fat is not bad; there are just some fats you should minimize in your diet and others you should make sure you include regularly. For optimum health, nutritionists recommend that we should get no more than 25 percent of our daily calories from fat and of that amount, no more than 10 percent should be saturated.

Saturated vs. Unsaturated Fats

Saturated fats are solid at room temperature, while unsaturated fats remain liquid under the same conditions. We have been taught for years that saturated fat is "bad" and unsaturated fat is "good," but as with most things involving the human body, it's a little more complex than that.

Saturated fats include products like lard and butter and unsaturated fats include products like olive and peanut oil. Unsaturated fats are classified either as monounsaturated, like olive oil, or polyunsaturated, like canola and sunflower oil.

While we tend to think that saturated fats come only from animal sources that is not true; coconut and palm oil are both saturated fats. To confuse the issue even more, not all animal fats are saturated. For example, beef has a bad reputation because we assume that all its fat is saturated. The majority of the fat in beef is actually unsaturated (42 percent vs. 38 percent saturated), and it includes fatty acids, like oleic and stearic acids, that may have beneficial health effects. Beef and many other animal protein sources also contain Conjugated Linoleic Acid or CLA, which investigators believe may inhibit tumor development. Because it contains so many nutrients, beef is actually an excellent food choice as long as it is eaten in moderation.

In nature, saturated and unsaturated fats occur in combination. For example, even a monounsaturated fat like olive oil, which nutritionists regard as one of the most healthful fats available, contains two grams of saturated fat per tablespoon.

We Need Cholesterol to Live

Cholesterol is another natural substance that has gotten an unfair reputation in recent years. Once researchers discovered it was the main component of arterial plaque, the waxy buildup known as atherosclerosis that can suddenly cut off blood flow to vital organs, they labeled cholesterol as public health enemy number one.

From the Medicine Chest

The USDA recommends we get no more than 300 milligrams of dietary cholesterol daily. Saturated fat intake should be less than 10 percent of our total caloric intake.

Cholesterol is so vital to our bodily functions that our livers actually manufacture it. It is used to build nerves and brain tissue and helps produce steroid hormones and the bile acids necessary for digestion. The problem is that our diets provide an excess of cholesterol. When we eat too many saturated fats, we are likely contributing to a buildup of excess cholesterol in our veins and arteries.

Trans Fats—the Real Villains

After World War II, many women who had gotten a taste of the working life found themselves reluctant to return to the role of full-time homemaker. As more and more women entered the work force on a full-time basis, the demand for prepackaged and easy-to-prepare foods skyrocketed.

Unfortunately, prepared foods tended to get rancid very quickly and had to be thrown away if not used in time. To reduce losses associated with spoilage, food manufacturers began casting about for ways to prolong the shelf life of their products. The first thing they did was to strip off the oil and essential fatty acid–containing outer husks of the wheat and rice grains they were packaging because this was the part that contained oil subject to rapid oxidation and spoilage. Without its protective and nutrient filled outer shells, wheat, and rice lasted much longer on grocery shelves.

Of course, they were much less nutritious as well, but at the time we weren't aware of all the health benefits we were throwing away along with the wheat and rice bran that we considered a worthless byproduct of the refining process.

Today, though many of us know better, consumers continue to snap up highly refined packaged products without stopping to consider the health consequences of eating a diet top heavy with convenience foods. As we explained in Chapter 5, researchers now believe the biggest culprit in our spiraling national epidemic of ill health and obesity is trans fat or hydrogenated oil, the cheap preservatives manufacturers use to extend the shelf life of their products even more.

Unfortunately, the products are ubiquitous in our American food supply with some researchers claiming that up to 90 percent of packaged and convenience foods contain hydrogenated oils, sometimes labeled as mono or diglycerides. These trans fats have been implicated in the development of everything from heart disease to breast cancer.

The problem is, our bodies don't know what to do with trans fats because they are artificial. So the body encases every molecule of trans fat it encounters with a protective coating of cholesterol and dumps it out of the bloodstream as quickly as possible. Depending on where the dumping occurs, you could be setting yourself up for a heart attack, stroke, impotence, pulmonary embolism, or blood clot in an extremity down the road—every molecule of trans fat that gets dumped narrows your arteries just a little more until one day they close up entirely, sealed off by a dam of gunk we have no business putting in our bodies at all.

Bottom line: *Read the labels*, and do your level best to completely eliminate trans fat in all its forms from your diet.

Essential Fatty Acids—the Good Guys

Ever wonder why they call essential fatty acids, or EFAs, essential? It's because they are essential; without them, life cannot be sustained. Yet when the "fat police" made their first sweep through the American diet about 15 years ago, they threw out the good fats with the bad. We now know that was a bad idea.

There are two essential fatty acids—Omega 3 and Omega 6. Our bodies cannot manufacture these vital fatty acids; they must be supplied either in our diets or through supplements.

Omega 9 is often confused with Omega 3 and 6, but while it is also vitally important to our health, it is classified as a nonessential fatty acid because our bodies can manufacture it in limited quantities. Omega 3 and 6 come from polyunsaturated fats, and Omega 9 comes from monounsaturated fats.

Omega 3 is found in heavy concentrations in brain cells; researchers believe it is a vital component in maintaining optimal functioning of the brain. One of the first signs of an Omega 3 deficiency is the development of mental fogginess and loss of ability to concentrate and stay on task. Omega 3 also makes blood platelets less sticky, reducing the risk of developing a blood clot.

EFA Name	Common Name	Good Sources
Omega 3	Linolenic acid (also called alpha-Linolenic acid)	Flaxseed, some nuts, canola, and soybean oils
	Eicosapentaenoic acid	Fish
	Docosahexainoic acid	Fish
Omega 6	Linoleic acid	Corn, safflower, soybean, cottonseed, and sunflower oils
	Arachadonic acid	Animal products
Omega 9	Oleic acid	Olive, peanut, and canola oils; animal products, including beef; and avocados

Omega 6 stimulates skin and hair growth, helps to regulate metabolism, and maintains reproductive and circulatory health. Food manufacturers add vegetable oils to almost all prepared foods, loading our diet with Omega 6s from corn, sunflower seeds, safflower seeds, cottonseed, and soybeans. This has changed the ratio of Omega 6 to Omega 3 fatty acids in our diet from the traditional range of 1 or 2:1 to approximately 20 to 30 to 1. This is too much of a good thing. Excessive amounts of Omega 6 in the bloodstream stimulate overproduction of prostaglandins, which create the sort of inflammatory response associated with arthritis and some other autoimmune disorders.

The typical American diet, high in Omega 6 and deficient in Omega 3, may be a contributing factor in our ever-increasing incidence of heart attack, high blood pressure, Type-II diabetes, rheumatoid arthritis, Crohn's disease, and chronic obstructive pulmonary disease. A high intake of Omega 6 fatty acids can also cause clotting, swelling, and constriction of arteries that can lead to heart attacks and other diseases.

The good news is that increasing the intake of Omega 3 fatty acids and reducing the intake of Omega 6 to bring the ratio back into a 1 to 1 or 2 to 1 balance can reverse these detrimental health changes. Increase your intake of whole grains, seeds, nuts, leafy greens, or fish to obtain the required amount of Omega 3, and reduce your intake of prepackaged and convenience foods containing Omega 6 to balance your ratios as recommended.

From the Medicine Chest

For a healthy heart, eat like you live on the Mediterranean. The typical Mediterranean diet produces one of the lowest rates of cardiovascular disease in the world. Nutritionists believe it is because people in Mediterranean countries consume large quantities of olive oil, a monounsaturated fat that has been shown to reduce the levels of LDL cholesterol and raise the levels of HDL cholesterol in the blood, as well as relatively low amounts of saturated fat.

Triglycerides—Fat or Sugar?

A few years ago, most of us had never even heard of triglycerides, and we certainly didn't have any idea what they did in our bodies. When fats enter our digestive systems, an enzyme called lipase breaks each molecule apart into glycerol (sugar) and fatty acids. Your body then reassembles these components into triglycerides, which is three molecules of fat attached to a backbone of glycerol. If you've eaten a reasonable meal, your body burns all the triglycerides it makes for fuel. If you've overindulged, the excess triglycerides are converted back to fat and stored on your thighs, hips, or stomach, depending upon your particular genetic pattern of fat distribution.

It is only recently that scientists have started to consider that triglycerides may in fact be a risk factor for heart disease, although there is still no agreement on this supposition. High plasma triglyceride levels do seem to make the blood more sluggish or likely to clot.

Triglyceride Reading	Rating
40 to 99 mg/dL	Normal
100 to 199 mg/dL	Increased risk of heart disease
More than 200 mg/dL	Dangerous risk of heart disease

Eating a healthier diet and adding regular exercise to your routine can manage high plasma triglyceride levels. They can be measured using the same blood sample drawn to test your cholesterol levels.

What Fats Do

The human body is made up of some 70 to 100 trillion cells, each encased in a soft, permeable fatty membrane that allows the cell to draw in the nutrients it needs and expel wastes. Essential fatty acids keep these membranes permeable, which, in turn, keep our cells healthy.

When we deprive our body of essential fatty acids, it repairs damage in these crucial membranes with other fats that cause the membranes to become rigid and impermeable. Cells trapped inside these membranes become sick because they cannot draw in nutrients or expel waste. Accumulate enough of these "sick" impaired cells in your body and you will get sick as well.

In addition to being a source of energy, fat is essential to the body's ability to metabolize the fat-soluble vitamins A, D, E, and K.

Symptoms of Too Little and Too Much Fat

You might think there could be no such thing as too little fat, but people who religiously eliminate almost every trace of fat from their diet suffer distinct symptoms due to a lack of essential fatty acids. Here are a few of the most serious:

- Dry skin and hair
- Excessive thirst
- Insomnia
- Fatigue
- Mental confusion
- Increased blood pressure
- Increased risk of heart disease

People who consume too much fat suffer from a more familiar list of complaints:

- Weight gain
- Gallstones
- Increased risk for some cancers like breast and colon
- Increased risk for coronary artery disease

The bottom line is that fats are essential for our bodies to run properly. You wouldn't run your car without oil in the engine, and you shouldn't try to run your body without fat. Be wise in your choices, make most of your selections from the mono- and poly-unsaturated fats, and try to limit your saturated fat intake. If you follow these suggestions, believe it or not, your dietary fat intake can actually make you more and not less healthy.

Carbohydrates—Complex Only, Please

These days, carbohydrates may be even more maligned than fats in our diets. Diets too dependent on refined or simple carbohydrates have been implicated in weight gain, obesity, and a tendency to develop diabetes. So when we say your diet should include 55 to 60 percent carbs, be aware that we aren't talking about donuts and Twinkies. We're talking about beans, whole-grain breads and cereals, fresh fruits, and vegetables. That's where your carbs should be coming from.

Complex carbohydrates include not only sugar but also starches and fiber. Simple carbohydrates are just sugars. Both provide glucose, your body's preferred fuel.

Athletes like carbohydrates because they require less oxygen to burn than either protein or fat, leaving them more energy to perform at their peak. Before major events, many athletes "load" carbohydrates by eating pasta or other carb-rich dishes to give their bodies an extra store of glucose for performance. In fact, just about all of us "load" carbs, but unlike athletes, we do not burn off the excess. We convert it to fat for energy storage.

Plenty of people swear that carbs make them fat, when in reality, it's all the stuff we pile on top of the carbs that does the damage. A whole medium potato contains but 90 calories and a typical slice of bread about 70 to 80. But by the time we add in 2 or 3 tablespoons of butter, sour cream, bacon bits, and cheese, a potato may have turned into a 500-calorie bomb with 23 grams of fat.

Don't Be So Refined—You Need Fiber

When carbohydrates are refined for the purpose of increasing their shelf life, much of their nutrient value is stripped away, leaving behind the white sugar, white flour, and white rice that are the bane of any dieter's existence. Nature intended carbohydrates to be a sort of roughage that speeds our digestion along. Refining removes fiber from carbohydrates, and that creates digestive problems.

This may sound odd, but fiber improves digestion because it is indigestible. Our bodies use fiber to push food through the digestive tract in a timely manner. Without fiber, food just sits there, causing miserable digestive symptoms like constipation and gas.

> **CAUTION** **911!**
>
> Like most other good things in life, you can get too much fiber. If your diet has been low in fiber and you suddenly decide to add a lot of it, be aware that you will probably experience intestinal cramps, bloating, and gas. You can avoid this by introducing fiber slowly, giving your body time to acclimate itself to your new, healthier eating habits.

Though it has no nutritive value, fiber is still an essential part of our nutritional needs. Many studies have indicated that people who eat high-fiber diets have lower rates of heart disease, cancer, obesity, and digestive upsets than people who eat more refined diets.

When you add fiber to your diet, it is especially important to be aware of your water intake. Dehydration is one of the biggest factors in chronic constipation. If you greatly increase your fiber intake without drinking a sufficient amount of water, you could be setting yourself up for significant gastrointestinal distress. Drink at least eight eight-ounce glasses daily to keep your intestinal system operating smoothly.

You could probably hope to go your entire life without being forced to know what ITT or Intestinal Transit Time is, but we're going to tell you anyway. From the time you swallow a bite until the moment you eliminate it is your ITT. Faster is better.

Health Notes

In a famous research study performed in the late 1970s, an anthropologist decided to study the ITTs of African tribesmen whose diets consisted primarily of foods that were high in fiber. He discovered the tribesmen had an average ITT of 12 to 14 hours.

Contrast that to the typical American who eats a diet loaded with refined carbohydrates and almost no fiber. Their ITT averages 48 to 72 hours and in some cases tested, the ITT was a full week!

You may be asking yourself, "So what's the big deal if my food lingers in my intestinal tract for a while longer than average?" It's simple—when food hangs out in your system for that long, your body wrings every ounce of caloric value from it. In other words, if you indulge in a loaded baked potato but also eat the fiber-rich skin, you might eliminate that potato in 24 hours, giving your body time to process and extract perhaps only 70 or 80 percent of the potato's caloric value. However, if that potato sits around for three or four days, by the time it leaves your system your body will have extracted every single calorie from it.

Select most of your carbs from unrefined choices, and your body will thank you.

The Glycemic Index—Fact or Fancy?

Many years ago, a couple of endocrinologists noticed that glucose levels rose rapidly following a meal high in carbohydrates. This rise signals the body to release insulin to process the sugar circulating in the blood, but it also signals the body to convert the excess sugars to fat for storage. The SugarBusters! diet made much of a glycemic index that categorizes foods according to how much glucose they release into the blood stream.

Recently, nutritionists have begun to question the value of the glycemic index as a tool in weight management. The glycemic values were obtained in labs and don't truly show how a food performs inside the body. The lab measurements do not take into account the food's fiber content or other nutritive factors that might greatly affect the way the body responds to the glucose stimulus of that particular food.

While the majority of your carbohydrate selections should have moderate sugar content, don't let the high glycemic index of an otherwise health-promoting food like carrots or bananas scare you away.

What Carbohydrates Do

Carbohydrates are the body's preferred fuel source. In fact, they are the only fuel source your brain and red blood cells can utilize. The big controversy over carbs results from the fact that they trigger the release of insulin in your bloodstream. Certain diet gurus maintain that this is automatically a bad thing, but insulin release only becomes problematic when the diet consists primarily of simple sugars and carbohydrates and contains very little of real nutritive value. We'll discuss this subject in greater detail in Chapter 8, "Sugarholics and Junk Food Junkies—Remaking the Diets of Full-Time Snackers."

People who have been following a high-protein, low- to no-carb diet for a long period of time may find themselves developing one or more symptoms of carbohydrate deficiency:

- Heightened sense of stress and tension
- Exaggerated reactions
- Loss of appetite
- Inability to concentrate
- Dehydration
- Lightheadedness, fainting

Too high an intake of carbohydrates, particularly simple carbs, can produce its own set of problems, including the following:

- Fluctuations in energy
- Fluctuations in blood sugar or low blood sugar
- Fatigue
- Weight gain
- Food cravings
- Frequent hunger
- Headaches
- Tooth decay

As with proteins and fats, you need to find the optimum balance of carbs for your diet by maintaining your food journal for at least two weeks.

Decide for Yourself

The important thing to remember is that you are the only one who can determine the best diet for yourself. You can read all the books you want and never find any agreement among them about the perfect balance between carbs, protein, and fat. Those authors don't know you like you know you, so learn to trust the signals your body gives you and follow your own best instincts when determining the best nutritional plan for you.

The Least You Need to Know

♦ While different people may have somewhat different requirements for protein and carbs, generally speaking, our nutritional needs fall within a predictable range.

♦ Proteins are our body's building blocks; a deficiency can have serious health consequences.

♦ Elimination of all fats is just as dangerous as eating too much fat.

♦ Carbohydrates are our body's preferred fuels.

Chapter 8

Sugarholics and Junk Food Junkies—Remaking the Diets of Full-Time Snackers

In This Chapter

- ◆ But I hate health food
- ◆ All junk food, all the time
- ◆ Targeting children who eat unhealthy food
- ◆ Surrounded by food but there's nothing to eat
- ◆ Stress snack attacks
- ◆ Mob behavior

Everywhere we turn, we find junk food—it dominates the shelves in our groceries, and it's the main item on the menu in most fast-food joints. It's even invaded the once hallowed bastion of our nation's school cafeterias as cash-strapped educators succumb to the siren song of big food industry bucks in exchange for allowing pizza chains and burger franchises to take over school food service.

In this hurried workaday world, we eat what we can easily get our hands on, and that usually means high-calorie; low-nutrient; fat-, salt-, and sugar-laden junk foods. We don't spend much time thinking about the health consequences of these poor choices, and that's a mistake. Talk to any doctor or health-care provider, and they will show you research suggesting that many of the most deadly illnesses they treat originate from poor dietary habits.

911!

In December 2000, the U.S. Department of Agriculture released a position paper titled "A Healthy, Well-Nourished Population." It stated: "4 of the top 10 causes of death in the United States are associated with diets that are too high in calories, total fat, saturated fat, or cholesterol, or too low in dietary fiber."

That means that many cases of the cardiovascular disease, Type II diabetes, and cancer could be prevented if people would simply pay more attention to the food they eat.

Need a harder number? How about government research that shows obesity and overweight contribute to 300,000 premature deaths every year? And as bad as that is, the number of premature deaths is only growing.

Even though most of us know better, we tend to avoid healthful eating. We have been led to believe that nutritious food doesn't taste good; that only snacks loaded with sugar, salt, and fat are worth having. Nothing could be farther from the truth. Think about it—the only difference between genuine artificial ranch flavor and genuine artificial teriyaki flavor is a few carbon molecules. Contrast this to the world of real food, where you have hundreds of seasonings from which to choose and many different methods available to prepare food.

Yes, healthy eating is something you have to think about and plan for, but once you get the hang of it, making wise food choices will become as natural to you as breathing. We promise. So read along as we help the sugarholics and junk food junkies among you remake your menus and boost your wellness in the process.

Health Food and Healthful Food—There Is a Difference

People complain that "health" food tastes awful, and for the most part, I'm inclined to agree. If I wanted to chew on cardboard, I could just grab a box; it would be a lot cheaper than these $2 and $3 "health" bars that are all tricked out with fancy names and packaging but still taste like raw cellulose.

So you won't catch me arguing that you have to invest huge sums in "health" food to enhance your wellness. But health*ful* food? Healthful food is inexpensive, it's quick and easy to prepare, there are hundreds of choices, and it tastes delicious. Yes, it really does. And once you get used to it, you won't ever want to touch another Twinkie again.

I know what you're thinking. This woman must be one of those nuts who puts bean sprouts on her bran flakes. Nope, I only put them in my salads. And I'm not preaching from some ivory tower. In the not too distant past, my nutritional choices were highly suspect. I wrote about health, wellness, and good nutrition all the time, but I never took any of my own advice.

The work area around my computer looked like the shelves in a convenience store—chips, cookies, gum, chocolate, hard candy, and in the refrigerator, enough ice cold soda to float the *Queen Mary*. Then I had a health scare, and that was enough to wake me up and make me examine my own eating habits. Now I preach and practice good nutrition with all the fervor of the true convert because I have seen the enemy, and it was in fact, me. Or maybe it was the seven-layer dip or the Ding-Dongs.

Wellness Words

It's telling that the term **junk food** did not enter our dictionaries until the year 1971. According to *Merriam-Webster*, it means: "food that is high in calories but low in nutritional content." The term has now been snagged by writers to indicate something that is appealing or enjoyable but of little or no real value.

Morning, Noon, and Midnight Munchies

Does this sound like you? You get up in the morning and grab two donuts and a mocha frappucino on the way to work. At 10, the coffee cart comes around and you buy another cup of joe, plus a candy bar and a bag of chips for later, and a blueberry streusel muffin to eat with your coffee.

At lunchtime, you go out with your friends to a nearby "all-you-can-eat" pizza parlor where you wash down four slices of pizza with two 36-ounce sodas. Because you are watching your weight, you split a piece of cheesecake with your friend for dessert. By 2 P.M. you're hungry again, so out come the chips and the candy bar, but they don't really do the trick so you go to the vending machine and get an iced apple pie.

Around three o'clock, you feel the familiar rumblings of indigestion. When reach into your desk drawer for some chewable antacids, you see a bag of cookies you've forgotten, so out they come and down the hatch they go. Of course, this makes you thirsty so you go to the drink machine but you feel bad because you realize you've been pigging out all day long, so you get a diet soda and then scurry guiltily back to your desk.

You have a late meeting, and on the way home, you go through a fast-food drive-thru because you are just too tired to cook. You order a double cheeseburger with special sauce, a chocolate milk shake, and then figure what the heck and you super-size your fries and soda. When you get home you are still hungry for something, so you grab a big bowl of ice cream slathered with Hershey's syrup and wolf down half a box of Double Stuff Oreos.

Your stomach starts to rumble again so you take a dose of Metamucil right before you go to bed and hope that will settle everything down. But your indigestion is so bad that you don't sleep well and when you wake up the next morning, you start the same routine all over again.

Congratulations. You have just taken in enough calories to sustain an entire Army platoon for one week. And you're not alone. Most of your friends at the office or in your apartment complex or down the block probably eat the same way every day. You are junk food junkies.

Before you start beating up on yourself, remember this fact—modern American life is not exactly conducive to healthful eating. It's natural for us to want to snack. In fact, many experts say it is better to eat five to seven small meals a day than three big ones.

Health Notes

Here's some good news. Frequent, healthy snacks may actually help boost your health. Researchers fed the exact same diet to two groups but divided the food differently. They fed one group of subjects 3 normal-size meals a day and the control group 17 healthy snacks spaced evenly over the course of the day. Despite the fact that the diets were identical in calories, fats, carbs, and protein, subjects fed the "snacking" diet showed significant decreases in their cholesterol and LDL cholesterol after two weeks. Researchers concluded that eating smaller, more frequent meals and snacks could lower heart disease risk as long as people were careful not to increase their overall caloric intake by eating more frequently.

The trouble is that most food readily available to us is not nutritious; in fact much of it is downright detrimental to our health. It's full of chemicals and additives that save manufacturers and grocers money because they cut down on spoilage but cost you money because they undermine your health.

Sometimes it seems as if our "nutritional plan" consists of nonstop bounding from one high-calorie, high-sugar, high-fat, and high-salt snack to another. It's no wonder. Look in our vending machines. Do you see anything remotely healthy in there? And do you see some things masquerading as healthy like "baked" chips and "low-fat" snacks that are nonetheless loaded with sugar and salt? So if you decide your health is important enough to make a change in your snacking habits, be aware that you'll have to plan and prepare your own snacks, because there won't be anything on the coffee cart or in the vending machine that supports the wellness lifestyle. Sure, it's a little extra work, but aren't you worth it?

Un-Happy Meals and Snacks

In many modern working families, the eating habits we just described are the stuff of daily life. When both Mom and Dad have full-time jobs, there is not much time left for meal planning and preparation, particularly in families with small children. But it's precisely in families with small children that meal planning is most important if we want to teach our children healthy eating habits and save them from the epidemic of obesity that is plaguing many adults and school age children today.

Health Notes

The National Restaurant Association says Americans eat out an average of four times a week for an annual total of 213 meals per person consumed at a restaurant or cafeteria. They spend almost 48 percent of their food budget on meals consumed outside the home.

Here are some more interesting restaurant facts:

◆ One in four retail outlets in this country is an eating or drinking establishment.

◆ Americans spend $878 million a day in restaurants—more on holidays.

◆ Nine million people are employed in the restaurant industry.

Food industry giants target children because they know how susceptible they are to suggestive advertising. The toys they offer with their "un-happy meals" are for the most part, truly intriguing. When tied in to a popular movie or toy phenomenon, the premiums seem irresistible to young children. And if you're the only mom and dad on the block who won't let your offspring get the genuine Disney Beanie Monster Duck Quacker, your child will probably grow up maladjusted and need years of therapy. At least that's what they'll tell you.

It's hard to stand up to the heartfelt supplications of your own kids, but if you love them (and we know you do), you will do it to protect their own health.

If your children really want the toys associated with a particular fast-food promotion, you can purchase them without subjecting your child to the high-fat meals that come with the toys. All the chains now sell the toys individually for very reasonable prices, usually $2 each. Purchase the toys and package "healthy meals" for use at home or on a picnic, and reward your child with the desired toy as a way of reinforcing good eating habits instead of the bad habits promoted by most fast-food meals.

A recent government report stated that fully 22 percent of children are clinically obese, with another 20 to 25 percent at least 15 percent over their ideal body weight. The problem is even worse for Hispanic and African American kids. The last time researchers checked (in the 1950s), it had taken more than 30 years for the number of obese kids to double in this country. This most recent poll indicates that the number of obese children has doubled in just the last 10 years and is expected to double again with the next 7 years unless immediate steps are taken to reverse the tide.

Experts point the finger in many directions:

◆ Harried working moms and dads have little time to prepare nutritious meals at home. They rely upon the convenience of take-out food, which is generally higher in fat and calories and lower in nutritive value than food prepared fresh at home.

◆ Instead of playing actively outside or engaging in after school sports activities, modern children lounge inside in front of TVs and computer terminals. They barely move except to push the buttons on the remote.

◆ Many schools have eliminated or greatly cut back on their physical education programs just at the time when our kids need regular exercise and physical activity the most to counteract the awful diets we are feeding them.

> **CAUTION**
>
> **911!**
>
> A February 2000 statewide survey showed that 71 percent of all schools in California serve fast food in place of more nutritious fare. If all your children's cafeteria offers is fast food, you should consider preparing healthy and appealing brown bag lunches for them to eat instead. To make sure they will eat what you send, make them part of the planning and preparation process.

Another real problem is the poor nutritional quality of the meals being served to many school children. The kind of junk food they get at lunch these days actually promotes weight gain.

My children's high school is typical. When my daughter was there four years ago, there was a salad bar and a cafeteria line serving balanced meals—not exactly gourmet fare, but not junk food either. Last year, the school was moved into a shiny new building, and my son discovered that all he could get for lunch was pizza because a major national pizza chain had taken over the food franchise in exchange for a large cash contribution to the school district.

Think about this: Day after day, week after week, all the children in this school may buy for lunch is pizza and soda. For variety they can switch back and forth from cheese to pepperoni, and if they really want to get fancy, they can order a supreme and get a few measly vegetables thrown into the bargain. How did we let this happen?

Well, for one thing, the parents weren't consulted. Their howls of protest after the fact had little effect other than getting cartons of milk added to the menu.

Our children deserve the very best food we can afford to give them. Take a close look at your life and your schedule and, if necessary, reorder some priorities to give you enough time to focus on healthful meal preparation. By starting your children off with healthful eating habits now, you'll be teaching them behaviors that will support lifelong wellness.

Food, Food Everywhere—but Nothing Good to Eat

Have you ever just stood in front of your open refrigerator or stared at a menu board in a restaurant until your eyes crossed, but you still couldn't think of anything that you really wanted to eat? One of the problems in a culture where food is abundant and cheap is that we often become bored with our meals. Part of the problem is that our bodies are much smarter about poor food choices than we are. They alert us with intestinal rumblings, headaches, fatigue, and other symptoms, but, for the most part, we ignore them. Finally, our brains play a trick on us—whenever we see a food that has given us problems in the past, even though we may not be consciously aware that it has, our brains send us a "not hungry" signal to keep us away from the culprit. When your diet consists mostly of junk food, your brain is layered with these "refusal" messages, which means you can literally stand in the middle of a huge grocery store and not be able to select anything that appeals to you.

This kind of apathy is due to one thing—boredom. Your body is bored with all the artificial foods you have been eating, foods that are so similar in composition and taste. It craves a healthy variety of fuels, and those "refusal" signals are one way that it tries to get it.

Those Helpful Folks in the Chem Labs

The food industry has been quick to fill the gap for busy people who think they don't have time to cook. Unfortunately, most of the products they produce contain unacceptably high levels of fat, sugar, and sodium and cost four to six times as much as the same type of food prepared from scratch. But many people keep right on eating the stuff, either because they don't know better or because there is really nothing else readily available that appeals to them.

Eating a balanced, nutritious diet that supports your health is simply a matter of planning and caring enough about yourself to only want the best for your body. But the planning can't start before the caring, or else your attempts to make positive changes will fail. You have to make the connection in your own mind between the constant consumption of junk food and poor health. You have to decide you are only going to put top-grade fuel into your "engine." Remember: good food = good health; poor food = poor health.

From the Medicine Chest

Among the top three causes of weight gain are poor food choices, reduced physical activity, and stress snacking. Certain medications may also cause weight gain. Counter these factors by planning for nutritious snacks and meals, increasing your physical activity to include at least three 30-minute exercise periods per week, and countering stress with a more beneficial method like deep breathing or meditation. If you think your medication is making you gain weight, ask your health-care provider if there is another medication available that will provide the same therapeutic benefits without the side effect of weight gain.

Does that mean if you eat a double cheeseburger you are going to keel over in the next 10 minutes? Of course not, but if cheeseburgers are a staple of your diet it does mean you are setting yourself up for eventual health problems. The damage caused by poor nutrition is cumulative; it may be years before you suffer some catastrophic event like a heart attack or stroke. But every bite of bad stuff you ingest is like a paving brick laying the foundation for health problems down the road. Keep laying those bricks, and sooner or later you will reap a harvest of ill health. Lay instead bricks of good nutrition, and the harvest you reap will be wellness.

It's Called an Apple

Sometimes we make things harder than they have to be. We reach for the applesauce when we could have had an apple. What's the difference? Plenty.

Food	Serving	Calories	Carbs	Sugar	Fiber
Applesauce	½ cup	110	27g	25g	2g
No-sugar-added applesauce	½ cup	50	13g	9g	2g
Apple, medium	1	80	22g	16g	5g

Not only are you getting higher calories and sugar in the half cup of applesauce, but you are getting a smaller portion size—about 122 grams as opposed to about 155 grams for the average medium-size apple. You're also losing something, namely three grams of pectin-rich fiber. That may not seem like much to you, but many studies have shown that a diet with adequate pectin (remember the old "apple a day?") actually lowers cholesterol.

If you really love applesauce, the healthiest choice is to select the no-sugar-added natural variety. You save 60 calories per serving over sweetened applesauce and eliminate 16 grams of sugar. You still don't get as many health benefits as you would from eating a fresh raw apple, but neither are you compromising your health by overloading your system with a big jolt of sugar like you would get from sweetened applesauce.

If you examine your diet, you will find many other places where you can make easy switches to save calories, sugar, and fat without sacrificing taste. As you slowly remake your diet, you will start feeling better physically and mentally and may even lose weight. You'll definitely save money.

Food	Serving	Calories	Carbs	Sugar	Fiber
Fresh raspberries	¾ cup	60	14g	7g	4g
Frozen raspberries	¾ cup	110	27g	25g	4g

Once again, the addition of sugar has turned a healthy natural food into something less desirable.

Keep Your Salads Healthy

Many of us like to grab a salad for lunch. While eating a meal composed of fresh raw vegetables seems like a healthy choice, the toppings we pile on at the salad bar or the additive-heavy packet of dressing that comes in prepackaged salads all serve to change a healthful food choice into a fat and calorie bomb.

One of the easiest ways to ensure your salads are healthy is to make your own dressing. You will have fresh, flavorful dressing in your choice of flavors for an entire week in exchange for an investment of about 10 minutes of your time every Sunday evening. Using your own dressing on a prepackaged grocery store salad not only saves you a few calories and greatly enhances the flavor of your salad, it also saves your body from the known and unknown effects of the chemical stabilizers, emulsifiers, and preservatives in store-bought dressings.

I counted the ingredients on a packet of "Lite" Buttermilk Ranch that came in a packaged salad I bought last week when I was on the run. There were 25. Number of ingredients in the delicious dressing I made myself and brought with me in a small plastic tub? Five— olive oil, freshly squeezed lemon juice, freshly minced garlic, brown mustard, and dried mint. If I can't pronounce it, I don't want it in my food.

It's incredibly easy to make your own delicious salad dressing. Just pour 1 tablespoon of good olive oil into a bowl or cup, squeeze in the juice of half a lemon, mince one or two cloves of garlic into the cup, and add 1 tablespoon of brown mustard and 1 tablespoon of dried mint. Whisk together with a fork and serve immediately or transfer to a small container to take to work or out to eat.

Food	Serving	Calories	Carbs	Sugar	Fiber
Dressing	2 Tbsp.	127g	4g	0g	14 g

This recipe is not that much lower in fat than bottled dressings—14 grams per serving as opposed to 17 or 18 grams for bottled—but you are skipping all the preservatives and getting the sort of great, fresh taste that never comes out of a bottle. Once you see how easy it is to make your own tasty dressings, you'll never go back to the bottled again.

In addition, most dressing packets list their serving size as "one pouch," cleverly disguising the fact that the "pouch" contains 44 milliliters or 3 full tablespoons of dressing, much more than you actually need to dress a big salad generously. One tablespoon is plenty if you toss the salad well; if you really must have more, limit it to two tablespoons. If you give in and add the entire "pouch," then you'll also be adding unnecessary calories and fat.

Are You a Chip Hound?

One of the most difficult snacks to give up is chips. Let's face it—giant manufacturers like Frito-Lay and Quaker spend millions of dollars annually developing and advertising new snack products. A successful recent entry into the field was chocolate-coated pretzels, popular because it combines three ruling passions—chocolate, salt, and crunch.

Chips come in so many intriguing flavors—ranch, mesquite BBQ, vinegar, rosemary and olive oil, sour cream and onion, cheddar—the list is endless. But all the flavors are the result of food chemists' wizardry; little derives from actual real food. But that "fakeness" makes them no less appealing, even though it should.

If chips are your weakness, try this technique. Whatever amount you are eating now, cut it in half. Substitute a healthy snack of your choice when you get the chip urge. After two weeks, cut your chip ration in half again, then two weeks later, cut it in half again. By this time, you should be down to no more than a few chips a day. The next time you bite into one, really think about it and see if it is starting to taste different to you. Using this regime, you should gradually lose your taste for chips over a period of about six weeks as you develop a taste for fresher food.

Once you have sharpened your taste buds by treating them to well-prepared fresh and healthful foods, you will discover you have a new zest for eating. You won't ever again stand in the middle of a store unable to decide what you want to eat.

Stress and Snacking

If your boss yells at you, do you reach for a Milky Way? If your little darling punches out another kid at the daycare center, do you fall back onto Fritos? If your significant other takes a hike in the middle of the night, do you console yourself with Häagen-Dazs and Chipperoos?

If so, you might be a stress snacker, someone who normally tries to eat a reasonable diet but who falls back on old, bad habits when the going gets tough. Like any other habit, stress snacking is a learned response. The best way to tackle it is to learn new, healthful habits to replace your automatic stress response of junk food snacking.

Try these techniques when you are upset and you feel the need to reach for an Almond Joy:

◆ Take 10, deep full breaths, inhaling through your nose until your lungs are completely expanded, then exhaling through your mouth. This technique gives your body the equivalent of an oxygen rush; the extra energy may serve to distract you from your desire to snack.

◆ Think of five healthy things you could have instead of the unhealthy snack you desire, then eat the one that most appeals to you. Savor it slowly, bite-by-bite over at least 20 minutes to give your body and your brain time to feel satisfied.

◆ If you are home, take a relaxing bath with aromatherapy salts or oil added to the tub. Select an oil like lavender or eucalyptus, known for their stress-reducing and calming properties.

Try to identify the people and situations that trigger stress eating. Once you admit you're addicted to sweet or salty snacks or both, make a firm determination to change. Keep track of these occasions in your food journal and note what you did to combat the urge to eat an unhealthy snack. Eventually, you will find that you are able to meet the urge to stress snack head on and replace it automatically with healthier behaviors.

Going with the Crowd–Following the Line of Least Resistance

Sometimes, even long after you have learned to make your snacking a health-building event, you will be confronted with a situation that makes you drop all your convictions and fall right back into the pit. The important thing is to be kind to yourself when this happens. You're only human and when you see people stampeding the buffet table at a wedding reception, it's natural for you to want to get right in there and fight with the best of them. As you are elbowing your way toward your fourth helping of Swedish meatballs, consider this: Catastrophic health events like stroke, heart attack, and gallstones are more likely to occur after people have gorged themselves with high-calorie, high-fat meals.

Here are a few strategies to help you manage your food intake when mob behavior threatens to take over:

◆ Just because it's a finger sandwich doesn't mean it's free of calories. Remember 3 finger sandwiches equal 1 regular sandwich, so if you have 12 of them on your plate, you are eating the equivalent of 4 sandwiches in one sitting. And that's not counting the petit fours or the cheese cubes or barbecued links or shrimp cocktail or roast beef roll-ups also on your plate. You would never eat this amount of food under normal circumstances, so there's no reason why you should eat it just because there's a wedding or a birthday or a retirement party. Moderation is the key.

◆ Eat slowly. If you wolf down your food, you will still feel hungry even after your stomach is completely filled with food. If you go back to the buffet and pile on more, your stomach will not be happy.

◆ If there are 10 things on the table that you absolutely must try, take just 1 or 2 bites of each. That will be enough to give you a taste without overloading the calories.

◆ Don't pile your food. Not only is it bad manners, but piling on is an open invitation to pigging out. Fill your plate with one layer of food and eat it slowly, then wait 20 minutes. If you truly still feel hungry, go back and select one additional item and eat that slowly until you feel the sense of satiety kicking in.

◆ If other people are shoving food at you, be polite but firm in telling them you have already had enough and don't want to eat anything more.

The Least You Need to Know

◆ You don't have to like health food to eat a healthful and nutritious diet.

◆ Diets consisting primarily of junk food promote ill health.

◆ Children are particularly vulnerable to the wiles of junk food marketers; it's up to us to teach them better eating habits.

◆ If nothing appeals to you, that might be a sign that your body is tired of junk food.

◆ Stress can trigger junk food cravings

◆ Even people who have good eating habits can be lured into overindulgence when they're in crowds.

Chapter 9

Planning Healthy Snacks and Meals

In This Chapter

- ◆ Planning is the key
- ◆ Smart shopping
- ◆ Easy cooking tips
- ◆ Super snacks and little brown bags

We often hear that one of the reasons fast food, packaged food, and eating in restaurants has become so popular is that men and women today are just too busy to cook. We understand; sometimes it seems like we're too busy to breathe, but the decision to cook nutritious, tasty meals at home is simply a matter of ordering your priorities and learning a few simple tricks to make cooking a full meal a breeze. In this chapter, we'll show you how it's done.

Smart Planning Makes Healthy Meals Easy

Nothing happens by accident, and that is certainly true for home-cooked meals. It definitely takes planning to make everything work smoothly.

Some people cringe at the mere idea of having to sit down and think about a meal three or four days before it is prepared. But taking a couple of hours a week to make a menu, write a grocery list, and then make one trip to the store can save you many more hours over the course of the week.

Include Your Family in the Planning Process

Sit down with your family on a convenient weekend day or evening with a calendar. Try to keep the time the same every week so that it becomes a family ritual. We suggest you include your family in the planning process for several reasons:

◆ Children will never learn how to prepare healthy meals and snacks unless you teach them.

◆ Putting together a trip to the grocery store involves many skills that children need to learn besides planning ahead—budgeting, time management, storage management, sensible food utilization, negotiation, and bargaining skills.

◆ Most moms and dads are already overly busy. By involving the entire family, the workload is shared, and the family gets a weekly opportunity to share time together while performing a job vital to the family's upkeep.

◆ Children who are involved from the start in the selection and planning of healthy meals feel proud and empowered when some of their choices make it onto the menu. They are more likely to be compliant with the family's improved eating habits and less likely to create problems or refuse new foods altogether. Best of all, they will be learning good eating habits that will last a lifetime.

◆ The family time will give you an opportunity to explain to your children (and to your spouse, if he or she is being childlike about trying new dishes) why you are making the changes and why they are so important to you and to the health of the family.

Making Lists

Discuss what you would like for breakfast, lunch, dinner, and snacks for each day of the coming week. Start your list as family members make suggestions. If your family already has a number of healthy dishes that they like, be sure to regularly include them on your menu.

Plan breakfast, lunch, and dinner for the entire week. Here's a sample dinner plan:

◆ Monday—stir-fried chicken and vegetables

◆ Tuesday—turkey chili with beans and cole slaw

◆ Wednesday—grilled chicken breasts with steamed mushrooms, rice, and broccoli

◆ Thursday—turkey burgers and green salad

◆ Friday—tuna casserole with vegetables and noodles

◆ Saturday—dinner out

◆ Sunday—roast beef with mashed potatoes and green beans

Compare the ingredients on your menu list with the items you already have in your pantry, freezer, and refrigerator. Then make a shopping list that contains the items you do not have on hand, plus any items that you'll need to restock after you finish your week's cooking. Notice that two dinners feature ground turkey and two others use chicken breasts. This type of planning makes it possible to buy larger quantities and take advantage of family-pack discount pricing.

Health Notes

According to a 1995 study commissioned by the U.S. Department of Agriculture and performed by Economic Research Service, 5.4 billion pounds of food were lost to waste or spoilage at the retail level in 1994, accounting for less than 2 percent of the available food supply. But when that same food found its way into the hands of consumers and food servers like restaurants, that loss rose to 91 billion pounds of food, meaning that almost 26 percent of the available food supply was wasted. The original 1994 food supply was estimated to provide 3,800 calories per day per person, more than $1\frac{1}{2}$ times the average person's daily energy needs.

Another advantage of menu planning is that it cuts down on overbuying, which in turn helps reduce waste. Americans purchase and consume much more food than people in any other part of the world, and we also waste more. We think nothing of spending $100 or more on a week's worth of groceries, then we throw half the stuff away because we overbought and it spoils before we can use it.

Once you have made your list, make a silent pledge that you will do your best to stick to it when you get to the grocery store. Every time you give in to the impulse to buy something not on your list, you spend more money than you budgeted and also increase the likelihood of something not-so-healthy sneaking into your basket.

With your list and determination firmly in hand, you are now ready to go to the store!

Smart Shopping

You may not know it, but grocery stores are laid out like mine fields, cleverly planted with little booby traps around every corner designed to blow you off budget. There is an entire industry devoted to the science of separating grocery shoppers from their hard-earned money. Gimmicky, high-profit impulse-buy items are always displayed on the end of aisles, where you will be most likely to see them and respond to the temptation they offer.

Staying the Course

Stick to your plan and you'll be fine. If you're worried about being tempted, give yourself a pair of figurative blinders and walk right by all the displays that are calling out to your fat cells.

Here are some proven tips to help you save money on groceries:

◆ Stick to your shopping list.

◆ Do not shop for groceries when you are feeling hungry; you will spend about 20 percent more than you had planned, often on unhealthful foods.

◆ Make the outer circuit of the store where the fresh fruits, vegetables, bread, meat, poultry, and fish are displayed and try to avoid the inner aisles except to replace staples like oil and vinegar. Why? Because, just like the end caps, the inner aisles are packed with items designed to encourage impulse buying.

◆ Leave your children and spouse at home, because if they tag along you will be much more likely to give in to the urge to impulse buy and overspend. Generally speaking, items bought on impulse are likely to be less healthful. If your spouse is the designated grocery shopper, keep the children home and let him or her shop alone and without distractions.

Now that you have whatever meat, dairy, and produce you need for the entire week, it's time to go home and do some prep work to make the week's cooking go smoothly. Shopping this way lets you get your entire week's groceries bought in one trip and also lets you take advantage of store sales to buy in bulk with no waste. The storage tips in the next section will greatly minimize food loss due to spoilage.

Putting It Away

You should have a workable kitchen space and a place for everything. The first thing to do when you return from the grocery is to put all your food away in its proper place. This may sound silly, but you'd be surprised at how much food is lost because a phone was ringing when a busy mom or dad came through the door with a sack of frozen food. By the time the call is over, the food might have melted all over the floor.

Tips and Tricks for Easy Cooking

As with most things in life, half the battle in cooking is your attitude. We promise you that absolutely anyone who can read a cookbook can prepare delicious meals. Our job is to show you how to maximize your time and productivity so that cooking actually becomes an enjoyable activity.

Organizing Menus and Recipes

Look at your week's menus and recipes and figure out how much work you can do ahead of time. In our experience, the smartest timesaver is to do most of your prep work on Sunday afternoon or evening; that makes cooking the rest of the week very easy.

Wash and dry your produce. Look at your recipes and determine which fresh vegetables are required and process them as necessary. For example, you might have sliced carrots on your Tuesday dinner menu with carrot slaw for a Thursday lunch. On Sunday afternoon, slice and vacuum-seal the raw carrots for Tuesday's dinner, then grate and vacuum-seal the raw carrots for Thursday's lunch. With a food processor and vacuum sealer, this entire operation will take no more than 5 to 10 minutes.

Repeat this process for all your fresh produce. If you have a vacuum sealer, you can do all the slicing and chopping for the entire week in an hour or so on one weekend afternoon. There will be no loss of taste or food quality, thanks to the vacuum-sealed pouches.

From the Medicine Chest

Weight Watchers has a comprehensive series of cookbooks containing recipes for a variety of family-pleasing dishes. Because there are no forbidden foods on this food plan, the meals do not seem like "diet food." If you only want to buy one cookbook, Weight Watchers publications are a good place to start. Your family might not even notice they are eating "healthy."

Next, divide your meat into meal-size portions, vacuum seal it in pouches, and freeze it for use later in the week. If one of your meals is burgers, take the time to shape the burgers before you freeze them.

Once you have all the ingredients for a particular meal prepared and packaged, put all the packages into a larger zip-lock bag and label it "Monday's dinner," or "Thursday's lunch." Take the meat for that meal out of the freezer the night before and put it in the package with the other ingredients. By the time you come home Monday evening, the meat will be defrosted and all you have to do is reach into the refrigerator, take out the Monday bag, fire up the stove, and dump in the prepared ingredients according to the recipe. Dinner will be ready in less than half an hour—just enough time for your kids or significant other to set the table and wash their hands.

Label each meat package according to the night it will be used. For example, if you are having burgers Tuesday night, label the pouch "Tuesday." When you finish the dishes Monday night, the last thing you should do before turning off the kitchen light is reach into the freezer and move the Tuesday pouch into the Tuesday meal bag in the refrigerator so that it may defrost overnight with no chance of spoilage. This way all your Tuesday meal ingredients will be grouped together and ready to go.

Assembling Your Ingredients

You've eliminated a lot of work by doing all the prep work on the weekend, but no matter how much work you do ahead of time, when you get ready to do the actual cooking, first you have to assemble your ingredients and your cooking utensils. For example, if your dinner is stir-fried chicken with Chinese vegetables, you have already cut up and vacuum-sealed your raw chicken breast strips and all your vegetables and you've got your wok set up on your stove. However, the recipe also calls for one tablespoon peanut oil, three tablespoons soy sauce, and one tablespoon cornstarch mixed in one cup water. If you start cooking before you have all this prepared, you can get into trouble quickly, particularly if you are cooking over high heat as is required for stir-frying. It's very easy to burn unattended ingredients while you are frantically searching for your cornstarch.

So before you even turn on the stove, make sure you have all the utensils, pots, and pans you need, as well as all the ingredients premeasured, premixed, and ready to go as soon as the recipe calls for them.

CAUTION

911!

Be careful not to give your children dangerous kitchen chores. For example, young children should never handle sharp knives or kitchen scissors, nor should they be anywhere near a hot stove with boiling pots. But they can easily handle plastic or metal measuring cups and love scooping and measuring flour, rice, and other dry ingredients. As they get older, they can graduate to measuring liquid ingredients. If they express an interest in cooking, consider enrolling them in a summer course at the YMCA or local community center. Once they reach the age of 12 or so, they are old enough to understand the basics of kitchen safety and can be allowed to use kitchen knives with supervision.

Just as you involved your family in the planning process, you should also get their help in the cooking process. Even very young children can be taught to measure properly. Have them measure out each ingredient such as herbs, salt, etc., and put each into a separate little dish. (We confess we got this idea from Martha Stewart, and it works really well.) Even if you are handling the cooking chores solo, don't skip this important part of preparation because cooking goes much more smoothly when you take the time to assemble all your utensils and ingredients before you start.

Familiarize yourself with some basic cooking terminology so that you may easily follow recipes.

- **Sauté**—fry in a very small amount of fat; sautéing is considered to be a more healthy way of cooking than frying
- **Poach**—cook in a simmering liquid; poaching can impart great flavor and tenderness to foods, particularly if the poaching liquid is a well-seasoned stock
- **Broil**—cook by direct exposure to radiant heat
- **Grill**—broil on a grill
- **Steam**—cook over boiling water in a closed pot
- **Braise**—cook slowly in a little fat and a little water or stock in a closed pot
- **Blanch**—scald in water
- **Sear**—seal by quickly exposing to intense direct heat
- **Roast**—cook in the dry heat of an oven
- **Fry**—cook over high heat by submersing in hot oil

You don't want to wait until you have a meal half-cooked to try and figure out what "braise" really means.

Cook Once, Eat Twice

One of the greatest timesavers for busy families is to cook more than one meal at a time.

For example, try cooking a double recipe of spaghetti sauce. Use half right away, and freeze the other half in a vacuum-sealed pouch for later use.

Try doubling the recipe for dishes like chili, casseroles, stews, and soups, then vacuum-sealing and freezing the extra portions for later use as a quick meal.

If your family likes hot oatmeal every morning but you don't really have time to cook it, make enough for the week on Sunday afternoon, then vacuum-seal it in individual serving pouches. The refrigerated pouches can be quickly reheated, and the oatmeal tastes as if it were just cooked fresh that morning.

If you like the taste of fresh bread, make enough dough on the weekend to meet your needs for the coming week. Shape it into loaves, rolls, pizza crusts, or whatever your menu plan requires. Then vacuum-seal the individual portions and freeze for use later in the week.

Clean Up as You Go

Sometimes people don't want to cook because they don't want to face a sink full of dirty dishes after the meal. With a few easy steps, you can make the cleanup process a lot easier.

Before you start cooking, draw a sink full of warm, soapy water and fill your second sink with tepid, clear water for rinsing. If you do not have a double sink, use a plastic dishpan for the soapy water and fill your sink with the rinse water.

As you finish using a utensil, pot, or dish, dip it into the soapy water and give it a quick wipe. Then dip it in the rinse water and put it on your dish drainer or into the dishwasher. If the item is stained or has food burned onto it, leave it sitting in the soapy water while you cook and serve your meal.

Relax and Enjoy Your Meal

Here comes the best part and the biggest payoff for the work and planning you have invested in your meals—enjoying them with your family and friends. All you have to do is relax and enjoy yourself. Don't rush. Eat slowly and savor every bite. Make dinner a time of pleasant conversation, exchanging tidbits of news with your family members. Mealtime can be one of the most important times of the day for families. Being part of a vibrant, loving, and happy family is one of the best ways to keep yourself well in the long run, and nothing can glue a family together like memorable family meals. You have all the tools at your disposal to start making those memories—now just do it.

Make Cleaning Up a Family Affair

After dinner, bring all your dishes to the sink. Remember to enlist the assistance of your family members. Scrape bones and other hard debris into the trash. Save soft scraps for your compost pile, put them in your garbage disposal, or simply throw them away.

Package and store leftovers. If you have a large quantity of leftovers, vacuum-seal and freeze them in a pouch. These pouches can be easily reheated by boiling or microwaving for a quick meal when you don't feel like cooking. Finish washing the pots you left soaking, then run the dishwasher if it is full. Finally, wipe down your stove and counters and remove garbage to the outside trash can.

These few steps can make your cleanup quick and easy. As you become more familiar and comfortable with cooking in this way, we're sure you will think up more timesaving ideas of your own.

Brownbagging Doesn't Have to Be Boring

Just as planning can help you tackle the job of cooking nutritious meals, so can it help you prepare healthy snacks and brownbag lunches. A little forethought can also help you negotiate a menu or buffet line when you are eating out.

Plan your weekly lunch menus at the same time that you prepare your grocery list. The ingredients for green salads can be prepared and packaged individually and labeled for the appropriate days just as you labeled your dinner packages. If you want your salad to be a meal, dice some turkey, ham, or cheese cubes to add protein. The dressing recipe in Chapter 8 can be prepared in less than five minutes. Make it the night before to allow the flavors to blend and store it in a small plastic container. Put the salad ingredients and the dressing in a larger storage bag and label it "Monday's lunch."

If you prefer sandwiches, assemble all the ingredients for the sandwich the night before—lettuce, sliced meat, tuna salad, etc., plus whatever sliced vegetables you desire like onions and tomatoes. In the morning before work, build the sandwich and package it. If you like mustard or a little mayonnaise on the sandwich, keep it in a little container and do not add it until you are ready to eat your lunch. This little trick will keep your bread from getting soggy and make your sandwich taste fresh.

Include whatever items you have chosen for your snacks in the bag, for example, sliced carrots with yogurt dip make a great snack, or you could select whole-wheat crackers with a couple of slices of low-fat cheese. Apples, oranges, and grapes make delicious choices.

Whole-grain, nonsweetened cereals are great substitutes for more fattening snacks. Bake in a low oven, 250°, for about 15 minutes on a cookie sheet lightly spritzed with oil and sprinkled with your favorite seasoning. Turn several times during the baking process, cool, and package half-cup servings in individual bags. Toss one into your lunch package for a tasty, crunchy, and healthy snack that won't break the calorie or fat gram bank.

If you like protein shakes, it takes no more than three or four minutes to make one in your blender each morning. Transfer it to a Thermos bottle and take it to the office. It will keep nicely even if no refrigeration is available. At 10 A.M., just as you are feeling an energy dip, you can reach for your protein shake, crackers and cheese, or fresh fruit instead of a doughnut, candy bar, or chips and soda.

In the morning, just grab your lunch and snack bag from the refrigerator, and you are ready to go.

From the Medicine Chest

If you don't like the idea of showing up at work with a literal "brown bag," there are several attractive and affordable adult "lunch box" systems available. Some have Thermos bottles; others have individual plastic containers meant to hold sandwiches and salads. Select whatever seems to best fit your needs, and pack your lunch in that.

Avoiding the Eating-Out Pitfalls

Sitting in a restaurant with a group of co-workers can be a real challenge for someone who is trying to remake their eating habits. Everyone wants to order the fried onion loaf appetizer and the greasy buffalo wings, and of course you need the three-quarter-pound burger, all topped off with a huge slice of New York cheesecake.

No one wants to stand out in a crowd, so here's the way to stick to your new nutritional standards while blending right in. Just about every restaurant menu now has "heart-healthy" choices. Look for those and try to make your selection from that portion of the menu.

If the menu doesn't offer heart-healthy selections, ask for a grilled chicken breast and green salad with the dressing on the side, which gives you control over how much dressing is added. Soups with clear bases like vegetable and onion soups also make good choices. Steer clear of cream-based soups that usually can harbor a lot of hidden fat. If you simply must have a burger, get a single and don't order all the high-fat additions like cheese and mayonnaise. A burger tastes pretty darned good with lettuce, tomatoes, onions, pickles, and a dab of brown mustard. You can save hundreds of calories and 30 or 40 grams of fat simply by making more thoughtful choices when you order.

If you love bread, skip the butter and ask for flavored olive oil to use as a dip. Don't ever give in and use the hard margarine generally supplied in restaurants. It's loaded with trans-fats.

Avoiding "All-You-Can-Eat" Pitfalls

There's something about human nature that makes us go wild when we see a buffet table loaded with tempting goodies. We take a bite of this, a spoonful of that, and before you know it, our plates are Leaning Towers of Pizza. We eat like there is no tomorrow, then an hour later we're groaning at our desks, suffering with heartburn, acid indigestion, and a variety of other unpleasant digestive complaints.

You *can* negotiate a buffet and still stay on your healthy eating plan. You just need a few smart tips.

First, watch your portion control. Fill your plate once, selecting one full portion of meat or two half portions. Add a couple of vegetables, preferably one orange or yellow and one green, and then a starch like noodles or potatoes. Skip the bread course if you want a bite of dessert.

Eat this amount of food slowly, chewing each bite thoroughly. Relax and enjoy the company you're with. If, at the end of 20 minutes, you still feel truly hungry, go back and get one more small helping of one dish and then stop there.

Keep reminding yourself we live in a civilized time and a civilized society. If your inner grunting Neanderthal makes an appearance at the buffet, simply escort him back to his cave and stick to your eating plan. With a bit of thought, you'll discover you can find something appealing *and* healthy on just about any menu or buffet table.

Life May Be Short, but Don't Eat Dessert First

Now on to the thorny subject of desserts. Cheesecake may be the single most tempting food on the face of the planet, but that still doesn't mean you should start every meal with a dish full of the stuff. Don't think: "Now that I am eating a healthier diet I can never again as long as I live enjoy a slice (or bite) of cheesecake." Think balance and moderation instead.

One way to tackle the dessert problem is to order one dessert for the entire table and then take one or two big, glorious bites and let your friends polish off the rest.

First, eat a nutritious, balanced meal, then eat that big bite of cheesecake. Take your time and savor it—even keep it in your mouth for five minutes if you have to. Just don't inhale it, because then you'll go back and eat the entire thing, including your friends' servings, your spouse's serving, *and* the slice you were saving for your great-aunt Betty.

Same thing with the hot fudge sundae, the apple pie, the double Dutch chocolate fudge layer cake, Mom's homemade brownies—all those tempting rich desserts we all love. Don't deny yourself, but don't eat the whole thing, either. Wait at least 20 minutes after the end of the meal for your "full" message to kick in and then enjoy a bite of dessert. You'll be much less likely to overindulge this way.

Finally, consider taking dessert the way the Europeans do, with a selection of fresh apples and pears along with a slice of cheese. It's light, refreshing, and healthy.

The Least You Need to Know

- Planning ahead will help you stick to your nutritional goals.
- Shop for groceries just once a week and you'll save time and money.
- Do most of your prep work on a weekend day and cooking during the week will be a breeze.
- Watch your menu selection and portion control when eating out.

Chapter 10

Vitamins—Do You Need Them or Not?

In This Chapter

- ◆ The discovery of vitamins
- ◆ Are vitamins really necessary?
- ◆ Fat-soluble vitamins
- ◆ Water-soluble vitamins

For centuries, people had no concept that the food they ate contained microscopic traces of elements vital to their good health. Nor did they understand that a lack of specific nutrients over an extended period of time could cause devastating disease and even death.

All that has changed. We now know that vitamins, minerals, and other trace nutrients are essential for human health. There's a growing interest in the use of herbs to support health as well. In this chapter we'll discuss how nourishing your body at the molecular level can help you stay well.

To facilitate ease of use, vitamins are listed in alphabetical order along with their benefits, best natural sources, symptoms of deficiency, potential side effects from overdose, and recommended daily intake for adults.

As with any of the information provided in this book, please consult your health-care provider before embarking upon a course of supplementation.

Certain vitamins can interfere with the action of prescription drugs; others may cause excess bleeding during surgery. Be sure to tell your doctor if you're taking any supplements so that he or she may be aware of possible interactions and conflicts with the protocols they're recommending.

One final note: In a perfect world it would be possible to supply all your body's nutritional needs simply by eating a balanced diet. We don't live in a perfect world. Much of our produce is grown on mineral-depleted soils, meaning that the fruit or vegetables harvested from such land contain lower-than-expected levels of nutrients. Our meat and poultry are contaminated with antibiotics, hormones, pesticides, and other undesirable chemicals, making it difficult to chart a course for eating well and staying healthy.

Because so much of our fresh food is nutrient-deficient, many health-care providers now recommend their patients take a daily multivitamin to ensure their health.

Vitamins—the Unseen Heroes of Health

Understanding only that the prescription worked, Egyptian physicians cured night blindness by advising their patients to eat foods rich in vitamin A, but this particular bit of wisdom was lost for centuries. Disease was attributed to angry gods or contagion; the idea that the lack of a specific food could make someone ill never came up.

British sailors spent long months at sea with little fresh food. Many developed scurvy, a deadly disease characterized by pain and spontaneous bleeding. It wasn't until 1747, when Scottish Naval surgeon James Lind discovered that including citrus in the diets of seafaring men eliminated scurvy, that an absolute connection was made between a nutritional deficiency and a disease. But Lind's advice was ignored for another 40 years while more than 100,000 additional British sailors died of the disease—more than had been lost in any war or at sea.

Someone finally stumbled upon Lind's research and acted upon it. Once the British provisioned their ships with crates of limes, the health and vigor of their sailors was restored. It might even be said that the nineteenth-century ascendancy and domination of the mighty British Naval fleet rested upon the tender branches of the humble lime tree.

From the Medicine Chest _____

Confused about which vitamins and minerals you need and how much of each you should take? No wonder. First there were RDAs or Recommended Daily Allowance for each vitamin and mineral; then the Food and Drug Association changed that to RDIs or Reference Daily Intake. Now the Food and Nutrition Board of the Institute of Medicine has established a new set of standards they call DRIs or Dietary Reference Intakes. For a comparison of the three standards, visit the Council for Responsible Nutrition at wwww.crnusa.org/Shellscire000002.html.

Once the idea that vitamins could cure or prevent disease was established, the rush was on to discover more vitamins and their uses. Scientists divided vitamins into two groups, fat-soluble and water-soluble. Research continues to this day. While we know much more about vitamins' role in our health than we did in the nineteenth century, we still have much to learn. Metabolically speaking, vitamins have diverse functions within our bodies, serving as precursors to the synthesis of other important substances, and also functioning as coenzymes, hormones, growth regulators, modulators, and antioxidants. They are the unseen heroes of our health.

Fat-Soluble Vitamins

The fat-soluble vitamins A, D, E, and K can't be absorbed and utilized by your body unless you take them with food that contains some fat. They bind with this fat, are absorbed through the intestines, and are stored in fat cells throughout your body.

Because your body stores fat-soluble vitamins and does not excrete excess amounts through the urine like it does with water-soluble vitamins, a real danger for toxicity exists when people take megadoses over an extended period. You should not take larger than recommended doses unless you are under the supervision of a health-care professional.

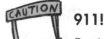

911!

Don't take megadoses of the fat-soluble vitamins A, D, E, and K. They are stored in body fat and can accumulate and reach toxic levels in your body. Taking large doses may cause severe and potentially deadly side effects. To be safe, stick to the dosage recommended by your health-care provider.

Vitamin A—Retinol

Vitamin A is made up of retinoids and carotenoids such as beta-carotene, a powerful antioxidant.

Benefits:

◆ Essential for good vision, especially night vision.

◆ Vital component in the growth and regulation of epithelial cells, which line the surfaces of the body.

◆ Helps body to repair damaged tissues.

◆ Enhances immune function; may protect against infection and the development of certain cancers.

◆ Helps to maintain healthy skin, bones, and hair.

Best natural sources—Yellow or orange fruits and vegetables, including carrots, sweet potatoes, tomatoes, apricots, peaches, cantaloupe, etc. Dark, green, leafy vegetables, including spinach, broccoli, kale, turnip greens, collards, etc. Also found in milk, cheddar cheese, egg yolks, and beef liver.

Symptoms of deficiency—Night blindness, dry, scaly skin, increased vulnerability to infection, loss of sense of taste.

Symptoms of overdose—50,000 IUs or more daily. Liver and nerve damage, nausea and vomiting, hair loss, headaches, loss of appetite, bone and joint pain.

RDI—5,000 IUs daily.

Vitamin D–the Sunshine Vitamin

Your skin can synthesize all the vitamin D your body needs as long as you get enough sunlight everyday. Vitamin D deficiencies may occur during the winter and where overcast weather is the norm.

Benefits:

- Controls absorption and utilization of calcium and phosphorus throughout the body.
- Builds strong teeth and bones.
- Helps to regulate cardiac function.
- Helps maintain a healthy central nervous system (CNS).

Best natural sources—Sunlight, eggs, yogurt, fatty fish like tuna, salmon, fortified foods like milk, and breakfast cereals.

Symptoms of deficiency—Bone demineralization or osteomalacia (softening of bones), resulting in bone pain and eventually, deformities. Accelerated tooth decay, inadequate absorption of calcium, muscle cramps, and poor healing of fractures.

Symptoms of overdose—25,000 IUs or more daily. Muscle weakness, calcification, or hardening of soft tissues in the body, including the heart and kidneys, headaches, excessive bleeding, and loss of appetite.

RDI—400 IUs daily.

Vitamin E

Researchers have identified eight distinct tocopherols or forms of vitamin E. Each plays its own unique role. Alpha-tocopherol is the form most often used by our bodies. Look for the natural form of the vitamin, which may include various combinations of d-alpha-, d-gamma-, d-delta-, and d-beta-tocopherols, and avoid the synthetic form, dl-alpha tocopherol or dl-alpha tocopheryl acetate.

Benefits:

◆ One of the most potent natural antioxidants, protects cells against damage from free radicals in the body.

◆ Essential component of reproductive health.

◆ Helps in formation of red blood cells.

◆ Helps to prevent degenerative diseases like arthritis, heart disease, and cancer.

Best natural sources—Nuts, seeds, legumes, whole grains, wheat germ, safflower and soybean oils, peanut butter, salmon, egg yolks, and green leafy vegetables.

Symptoms of deficiency—Because of the relatively high fat content of most American diets, vitamin E deficiency is almost unheard of in this country. Here are symptoms to look for: dry skin, hemolytic anemia, impotence, infertility, abnormal fat deposits in the muscles, muscular weakness, degenerative changes in the heart muscle, easy bruising, and slow wound healing.

Symptoms of overdose—3,000 IU or more daily. Inhibits clotting of blood and can lead to hemorrhage if injured.

RDI—50 to 400 IU daily.

Vitamin K—Menadione

Your body manufactures about 80 percent of the vitamin K it needs using special bacteria in the large intestine. Taking antibiotics wipes out these beneficial bacteria, so be sure to replace them with a product like Lactinex or you may suffer a vitamin K deficiency.

Benefits:

◆ Essential in the formation of blood-clotting proteins.

◆ Prevents calcification of soft tissues like arteries.

◆ Helps in formation of red blood cells.

◆ Promotes bone mineralization and repair.

◆ Helps regulate blood sugar.

◆ Assists in converting glucose to glycogen for storage.

Best natural sources—Green leafy vegetables like spinach, broccoli, green cabbage, cauliflower, alfalfa, legumes, whole-grain cereals, soybeans, strawberries, oranges, milk, and yogurt.

Symptoms of deficiency—Nosebleeds, internal hemorrhaging, slow clotting of cuts, bruising, and diarrhea.

Symptoms of overdose—Dosage not set. Extremely high intake can cause Hemolytic anemia.

RDI—65 to 80 mcg daily.

Water-Soluble Vitamins

Water-soluble vitamins include members of the B complex family and vitamin C. With the exception of B-12, which is stored in the liver, water-soluble vitamins are not stored in large quantities in the body. It is necessary to replenish your stores on an ongoing basis to maintain good health.

When you take too large a dose of a water-soluble vitamin, your body excretes the excess in your urine. However, megadoses can cause problems, so be sure to follow the dosage recommendations of your health-care provider.

From the Medicine Chest

The discovery of vitamins launched a scientific gold rush. Throughout the late nineteenth and early twentieth centuries, researchers discovered one vitamin after another. So many labs were working on similar research that several "discovered" the same B vitamin at almost the same time, labeling their find with the next number in the B vitamin numerical order. Once it was discovered that several labs had claimed the same B vitamin, the extra numbers were quietly dropped. That's why B vitamins jump from B-1 to B-12 with so many gaps in between.

B vitamins exist in particular relationships to each other. For example, B-9, folic acid, and B-12, cobalamin, work together to produce and regulate red blood cells. A deficiency of either one can produce a dangerous type of anemia. Most good supplements are formulated with appropriate amounts of B complex and other vitamins to maximize absorption and utilization by your body.

Cooking greatly diminishes the vitamin content of food, so including some raw food in your diet every day is important to maintaining good health.

Vitamin B-1—Thiamine

Benefits:

- Enhances circulation.
- Assists with carbohydrate metabolism.
- Essential for health of nervous system.
- Helps in manufacture of blood cells.
- Essential to manufacture of hydrochloric acid necessary for digestion.
- Plays a role in the biosynthesis of neurotransmitters.

Best natural sources—Whole grains, beef liver, pork, fish, egg yolks, peanuts, yeast, seafood, legumes, and wheat bran.

Symptoms of deficiency—Numbness in the hands and feet, extreme fatigue, irritability, nervousness, shortness of breath, palpitations, constipation, edema, forgetfulness, loss of appetite, and unexplained weight loss. Severe deficiency can cause a disease called beri-beri, heart failure, and death.

Symptoms of overdose—No limits set. No symptoms noted.

RDI—1.5 mg.

Vitamin B-2—Riboflavin

Benefits:

- Plays a crucial role in metabolizing carbohydrates, fats, and proteins.
- Boosts immunity by maintaining antibody reserves.
- Essential in the production of red blood cells.
- Helps with general tissue repair and speeds healing.
- Maintains central nervous system.

Best natural sources—Organ meats, nuts, cheese, eggs, milk, lean meats, leafy green vegetables, fish, legumes, whole grains, and yogurt.

Symptoms of deficiency—Sore throat; sores at the corners of the mouth; cracked lips; swollen tongue; weeping dermatitis; migraine headaches; itchy eyes; flaking skin around eyebrows, nose and earlobes; anemia; fatigue; and sensitivity to light.

911!

Don't take B-2 with alcoholic beverages. Alcohol keeps your intestines from absorbing riboflavin normally. That's why so many heavy drinkers have severe B-2 deficiencies.

Symptoms of overdose—No limits set. Harmless yellow-orange or bright yellow discoloration of urine with high dosage.

RDI—1.6 mg daily for men, 1.2 mg for women. Most supplements contain 50 mg, which is considered a safe dosage.

Vitamin B-3—Niacin or Nicotinic Acid

Benefits:

- ◆ Regulates cholesterol.
- ◆ Helps regulate blood sugar levels.
- ◆ Helps metabolize carbohydrates, fats, and proteins.
- ◆ Improves circulation.
- ◆ Relieves depression and anxiety and enhances mood.
- ◆ Reduces inflammation.

Best natural sources—Liver, tuna, chicken, salmon, nuts, lean beef, brown rice, legumes, and oysters.

Symptoms of deficiency—Pellagra, a skin condition characterized by patches of dry, itchy skin. Loss of appetite, general weakness, headaches, memory loss, depression, indigestion, canker sores, bad breath, and low blood sugar.

Symptoms of overdose—More than 100 mg daily. Flushing, liver dysfunction, nausea, stomach cramps, gout, dizziness, itching, low blood pressure, ulcers, and elevated blood sugar.

RDI—16 mg daily for men, 14 mg for women.

Vitamin B-5—Pantothenic Acid

Benefits:

- ◆ Supports adrenal gland.
- ◆ Essential in synthesis of hormones.
- ◆ Helps metabolize fats, proteins, and carbohydrates.
- ◆ Used to synthesize lipids, red blood cells, neurotransmitters, and steroid hormones.

Best natural sources—Beef liver, eggs, avocados, mushrooms, bananas, oranges, soybeans, potatoes, broccoli, whole grains, milk, legumes, and saltwater fish.

Symptoms of deficiency—Headache, tingling hands, fatigue, numbness, disturbed sleep, irritability, and infertility.

Symptoms of overdose—1,500 mg or more daily. Sensitive teeth—10 g or more daily. Diarrhea, bloating.

RDI—7 mg daily for men, 4 mg daily for women. May safely take up to 100 mg daily without adverse effects.

Vitamin B-6—Pyridoxine

Benefits:

- Aids in synthesis of antibodies and hormones.
- Regulates sodium and potassium.
- Assists in metabolism of proteins, fats, and carbohydrates. Requirements increase with additional protein intake.
- Supports healthy skin.
- Promotes normal brain function.
- Regulates hormones in women.
- Essential for proper function of enzymes.

Best natural sources—Bananas, watermelon, salmon, chicken, pork, potatoes, soybeans, tuna, brown rice, legumes, and spinach.

Symptoms of deficiency—Irritability, nervousness, kidney stones, acne, dermatitis, insomnia, and inflamed tongue.

Symptoms of overdose—More than 100 mg daily. Progressive permanent neurological damage, including sensory neuropathy, weakness, numbness, and ataxia, or the inability to coordinate movement.

RDI—20 mg per day.

Vitamin B-9—Folic Acid

Benefits:

- Regulates cell division and growth.
- Prevents neural tube birth defects.
- Essential in formation of red blood cells.
- Crucial for oxygen transport in blood.
- Assists in synthesis of amino acids.
- Coenzyme for RNA and DNA synthesis.

- ◆ Aids digestion.
- ◆ Promotes healthy nervous system.

Best natural sources—Oatmeal, fresh green vegetables like spinach and broccoli, lentils, legumes, whole grains, liver, and orange juice.

Symptoms of deficiency—Acne, sore tongue, fatigue, cracks at the corners of the mouth, anemia, osteoporosis, and depression.

Symptoms of overdose—More than 1 mg daily. Insomnia, digestive upsets, and intolerance to gluten.

RDI—400 mcg daily.

Vitamin B-12—Cobalamin

Benefits:

- ◆ Maintains protective myelin coating on spinal cord, optic nerve, and peripheral nerves throughout the body.
- ◆ Synthesizes RNA and DNA.
- ◆ Regulates homocysteine.
- ◆ Assists in metabolism of fat and protein.
- ◆ Manufactures and maintains red blood cells.
- ◆ Stimulates appetite.

Best natural sources—Lean beef, liver, chicken, shellfish, tuna, salmon, cheese, raw eggs, and dairy products.

Symptoms of deficiency—Back pain, sore tongue, apathy, erosion of the myelin sheath that protects nerves, pernicious anemia, loss of balance, ringing in the ears, decreased reflexes, and toxic buildup of homocysteine in the blood.

Symptoms of overdose—No upper limit set for oral dosage. Skin problems possible with too large a dose of injectible B-12.

RDI—3 mcg daily.

Choline

Benefits:

- ◆ Helps control weight.
- ◆ Regulates cholesterol levels.

- Prevents gallstones.
- Fights infections.
- Critical for normal membrane structure.

Best natural sources—Nuts, lean beef, oatmeal, wheat germ, and egg yolks.

Symptoms of deficiency—High blood pressure, elevated cholesterol, liver disease, inability to digest fats, fatty buildup in liver, liver disease, gallstones, and kidney problems.

Symptoms of overdose—More than 3.5 g daily. Depression, nausea, fishy body odor, low blood pressure, sweating, and diarrhea.

RDI—550 mg daily for men, 425 mg for women.

Inositol

Benefits:

- Helps cell membranes to function properly.
- Regulates estrogen levels.
- Promotes healthy hair.

Best natural sources—Bananas, liver, brown rice, brewers yeast, molasses, nuts, raisins, oats.

Symptoms of deficiency—Eczema, hair loss, constipation, vision problems, elevated cholesterol.

Symptoms of overdose—No upper limits set. Extremely high dose may cause diarrhea.

RDI—100 mg daily.

Biotin–Vitamin H

Benefits:

- Plays a vital role in the Krebs cycle, whereby energy is released from food for use in the body.
- Assists in production of fatty acids.
- Promotes healthy hair and skin.
- Helps regulate blood sugar.
- Assists in a variety of metabolic chemical conversions.

Best natural sources—Oatmeal, cottage cheese, salmon, soybeans, liver, yeast, eggs, milk, mushrooms, and bananas.

Symptoms of deficiency—Nausea, vomiting, loss of appetite, depression, swollen tongue, skin inflammation and dryness, hair loss, and elevated cholesterol.

Symptoms of overdose—No upper limits set. No symptoms of toxicity noted.

RDI—30 mcg daily.

Vitamin C–Ascorbic Acid

Benefits:

◆ Required to synthesize collagen, neurotransmitters, and steroid hormones.

◆ Assists in iron and calcium absorption in body.

◆ Antioxidant, protects against pollutants.

◆ Essential for normal tissue growth and repair, plus repair of wounds and burns.

◆ Strengthens capillary walls.

◆ Prevents bruising and blood clots.

◆ Helps to maintain healthy gums.

Best natural sources—Citrus fruit, berries, tomatoes, orange juice, cantaloupe, papaya, broccoli, and turnip greens.

Symptoms of deficiency—Bleeding gums, easy bruising, slow healing of wounds, swelling, poor digestion, decreased immunity resulting in more colds and upper-respiratory infections, painful joints, and general fatigue and weakness.

Symptoms of overdose—More than 2,000 daily may be toxic, but individual tolerance varies widely. The first sign of too much vitamin C is digestive upset with diarrhea, abdominal cramps, and bloating. Other risks may include kidney stones and increased iron absorption with excess stored in heart and liver.

RDI—90 mg daily for men, 75 mg daily for women.

The Least You Need to Know

◆ It took thousands of years before the connection between vitamins and good health was established.

◆ Vitamins are classified as water-soluble and fat-soluble.

◆ You can get too much of a good thing; overdosing on certain vitamins can cause severe side effects.

Minerals, Herbs, and Phytonutrients

In This Chapter

- ◆ Major minerals—small but mighty
- ◆ Trace minerals—you need these, too
- ◆ Herbs—more powerful than you think
- ◆ Phytonutrients—the newest player

Sometimes people who are good about taking vitamin supplements regularly completely overlook their body's mineral requirements. Minerals play many vital roles in running our bodies and are essential to continued good health.

You can tell something has entered mainstream culture when it shows up in formulations manufactured by major pharmaceutical companies. After spending some time out of favor, herbs have taken center stage in recent years. But the assumption that herbs are automatically safe because they are all-natural and plant-based can be dangerous. Herbs can be an extremely valuable addition to any wellness regimen, but just as with any other thing we take into our bodies, the use of herbs must be governed by moderation and thoughtful planning.

The newest player on the nutritional supplement team is phytonutrients, food-based nutritional products that are believed to reduce the risk of developing the degenerative diseases associated with aging.

In this chapter, we'll give you an overview of minerals, herbs, and phytonutrients and help you decide which ones are for you. As with any other supplement, consult your health-care provider before launching on any new regimen. Follow package instructions for dosing, and don't take more than the recommended amount. Finally, be aware that it is possible for many supplements, no matter how beneficial, to produce underdesirable side effects when taken in combination with other drugs or supplements. Well-controlled studies about the effects and side effects of herbs and supplements are not as plentiful as those for mainstream medical pharmaceuticals, and, thus, you should take these substances with care.

Major Minerals

Minerals are actually elements, fundamental substances that play many vital roles in the functioning of the human body. Minerals are part of our earth, swirling in our groundwater and taken up by growing plants. The only way we can get them is by eating food that contains them or by taking supplements. The mineral content of food is not consistent, because the mineral composition of soil varies dramatically by geographic region. To compensate for this uncertainty, it has become popular in recent years to add minerals to multivitamin formulas as a way to ensure that minimum daily requirements are met. Minerals must be taken together in precisely balanced formulas to ensure proper absorption, or deficiencies may result. If you are taking individual mineral supplements, ask your health-care provider to review your dosage to make sure you are getting everything you need to keep your mineral intake properly balanced.

Here's an overview of some of the most important minerals.

Calcium

Calcium is the most common mineral in the human body. There are five distinct types of calcium—calcium carbonate, calcium phosphate, calcium citrate, calcium lactate, and calcium gluconate. Each contains a different amount of the mineral. Read the labels on your supplements and antacids carefully. Calcium lactate and citrate are more readily absorbed and utilized by your body than the other kinds of calcium.

Benefits—The functions of calcium are so vital that your body will demineralize your bones to ensure you have an adequate supply. A list of all its functions could take several pages. Here are a few of the most important:

- Maintains bone structure and strength, repairs bone damage
- Intracellular messenger sends electrical signals to muscle and nerve cells
- Vital for blood coagulation
- Plays an essential role in the regulation of proteins and enzymes
- Maintains and repairs cell membranes
- Maintains regular heartbeat
- Exerts a calming and tranquilizing effect on the central nervous system

Best natural sources—Yogurt, milk, cheese, and calcium-fortified foods. Calcium from oxalate-rich, dark, green, leafy vegetables like spinach is poorly absorbed.

Symptoms of deficiency—Osteoporosis, increased risk of high blood pressure, heart palpitations, brittle nails, insomnia, muscle cramps, elevated cholesterol, eczema, and nervousness.

Symptoms of overdose—More than 2,500 mg daily. Possible kidney stones, irritability, headaches, constipation, and kidney failure.

RDI—1,000 mg daily under 50 years of age, 1,200 mg daily for people 51 and older.

> **CAUTION 911!**
> Watch your calcium intake carefully to make sure you don't get a toxic dose. Calcium is currently the *mineral du jour*. Its role as a media darling means food manufacturers are rushing to put it into everything from orange juice to breakfast cereal to candy bars. According to the USDA, 10 percent of Americans get too much calcium, and that can lead to health problems, too.

Phosphorus

At any given moment your body contains just 400 to 500 g of phosphorus, but without it, your body couldn't function.

Benefits—

- Helps convert food to energy
- Essential to kidney functioning
- Helps form and maintain bones and teeth
- Assists in storing and transmitting genetic information
- Assists in binding hemoglobin to red blood cells and in oxygen delivery throughout the body
- Regulates acid-base balance in body
- Regulates cell metabolism

Best natural sources—Bran cereal, almonds, American cheese, lean beef, pinto beans, shrimp, oatmeal, milk, and eggs.

Symptoms of deficiency—Bone loss and pain, fatigue, anemia, weakness, loss of appetite, depressed immune system, difficulty walking, and tingling in extremities.

Symptoms of overdose—More than 4,000 mg daily for adults up to age 70; more than 3,000 mg daily for adults over age 70. Calcification of soft tissues, particularly the kidneys, interference with calcium absorption, low serum and calcium levels, and calcium in urine.

RDI—700 mg daily for adults.

Magnesium

Magnesium regulates more than 300 essential metabolic reactions in your body. People with impaired kidney function must be careful not to get too much magnesium because of potentially life-threatening side effects.

Benefits—

- Assists in the absorption of calcium and potassium
- Relaxes muscles
- Transmits nerve impulses to muscles
- Helps regulate blood pressure
- Helps convert fats and protein to energy
- Helps synthesize RNA and DNA
- Transports ions across cell membranes
- An essential component of bone, cell membranes, and chromosomes

Best natural sources—Wheat bran, legumes, meat, bananas, milk, almonds, peanut butter, nuts, and dark green leafy vegetables.

Symptoms of deficiency—Abnormal heart rhythm, seizures, tremor, muscle spasms and weakness, nausea, and irritability.

Symptoms of overdose—More than 350 mg daily. Low blood pressure, muscle weakness, lethargy, confusion, deterioration of kidney function, sweating, slurred speech, difficulty breathing, and cardiac arrest.

RDI—400 to 420 mg daily for men, 310 to 320 milligrams daily for women.

Sodium

Sodium is nothing more than good, old-fashioned salt. Like the other major minerals, it is essential for life. Our diets provide an overabundance of sodium because processed and canned foods contain such high amounts.

Benefits—

♦ Helps maintain acid-base balance in body

♦ Vital for production of hydrochloric acid in the stomach

♦ Essential to maintain blood volume and regulate blood pressure

♦ Regulates water content in cells

♦ Serves as one of the body's most important electrolytes

Best natural sources—Table salt, soy sauce, cheese, cured meats, and seaweed.

Symptoms of deficiency—Diarrhea, vomiting, sweating, dizziness, weakness, poor concentration, disorientation, muscle cramps, and fainting.

Symptoms of overdose—More than 2,400 mg daily. Fluid retention and high blood pressure.

RDI—500 mg daily, more during hot weather when you sweat profusely, or if you are an athlete.

From the Medicine Chest

According to the U.S. Department of Agriculture, fully 75 percent of the salt that Americans get in their diets comes from salt added during food processing or manufacturing, rather than from salt added at the table or during cooking. If you want to lower your salt intake, you don't have to put away the saltshaker. Simply build your diet around unprocessed foods, with lots of vegetables, fruit, and legumes, and try to avoid prepackaged and highly processed foods and snacks whenever possible.

Potassium

Potassium is an electrolyte that works with sodium in many vital body processes.

Benefits—

♦ Works with sodium to transmit nerve impulses for the central nervous system

♦ Regulates muscle contraction

♦ Helps regulate heartbeat

♦ Helps build muscles

Best natural sources—Fresh fruits, especially citrus fruit and bananas, fresh vegetables, whole grains, molasses, fish, and lean meats.

Symptoms of deficiency—Fatigue, acne, muscle weakness, drowsiness, dry skin, mood swings, slow reflexes, mental confusion, and irregular heartbeat.

Symptoms of overdose—More than 4,500 mg daily. Irregular heartbeat, and cardiac arrest.

RDI—3,500 mg daily.

Trace Minerals–a Little Dab Will Do You

In addition to the major minerals previously listed, there are many trace minerals that your body needs as well. The requirements for these trace minerals may seem miniscule, but remember if your body doesn't get them, your health will suffer. No upper limit has been set for oral dosages of several trace minerals, indicated in the following information as "No UL." Even though there has been no recorded evidence of toxicity from a high oral dose of these minerals, follow RDI guidelines to ensure safety.

Chromium—Helps regulate the metabolism of sugar and fats and also helps regulate the amount of glucose in your bloodstream. Insulin won't work as intended in the absence of chromium. Deficiencies raise the level of insulin circulating in your blood and lower your glucose tolerance. No UL.

Best natural sources—Vegetables, especially spinach, mushrooms, apples and other fruit, peanut butter, and chicken.

RDI—50 to 200 mcg daily for adults.

Copper—Helps form red blood cells, helps the body absorb iron properly, and helps enzymes do their jobs. Deficiencies can cause anemia, neurological damage, and loss of pigment in the skin and hair. No UL.

Best natural sources—Beef liver, spring water, shellfish, legumes, nuts, and whole grains.

RDI—1.5 to 3 mg daily for adults.

Fluoride—Helps form bones and teeth and helps prevent cavities. Deficiencies may contribute to increased tooth decay and bone loss through demineralization of the bones. Although there is no UL for fluoride, overdoses can permanently discolor teeth and may impair kidney function.

Best natural sources—Fluoridated drinking water and seafood.

RDI—3.8 mg daily for males; 3.1 mg daily for females.

Iodine—Helps regulate metabolism and aids in proper development of fetuses. Deficiencies may produce a condition called goiter, which is an enlargement of the thyroid gland at the base of your throat. Deficiencies during pregnancy or early childhood may result in mental retardation and stunted growth. Although there is no set upper limit for iodine intake, overdoses depress the activity of the thyroid gland.

Best natural sources—Iodized table salt and seafood.

RDI—150 mcg daily for adults.

Iron—An essential workhorse in our bodies, iron is vital for the formation of hemoglobin, the part of our blood that carried oxygen in our blood and for myoglobin, which carries oxygen to our muscles. Iron also helps maintain a strong immune system. Iron deficiency is considered the most common nutrient deficiency in America. Deficiencies may result in anemia, pale skin color, depressed immunity, and fatigue. Too much iron can be dangerous, even potentially deadly. Although rare in the United States, toxicity can result from overconsumption of iron supplements, producing a condition called hemochromatosis, which can cause multiple organ failure and death if untreated. There is no UL established.

Best natural sources—Beef, eggs, poultry, legumes, dried fruit, dark green leafy vegetables, and anything cooked in iron pots.

RDI—8 mg daily for adult males; 15 mg daily for females.

Zinc—An essential catalyst for more than 100 enzyme reactions within our bodies, zinc is vital in the manufacture of protein and genetic material, stimulates hair growth, helps transport vitamin A throughout the body, heals wounds, is a vital component of our ability to taste, boosts immunity, and facilitates hormonal activity. Deficiencies lead to a loss of taste, poor wound healing, skin rashes, night blindness, stunted growth, and delayed neurological and sexual development in children. Doses of more than 100 mg daily can lead to abdominal pain, vomiting, diarrhea, and a copper deficiency.

Best natural sources—Shellfish, lean beef, eggs, nuts, and legumes.

RDI—11 mg daily for males, 8 mg daily for females, more if taking supplemental calcium or iron, as both of these minerals inhibit zinc utilization in the body.

Selenium—Selenium acts as an antioxidant within the body, boosts immunity, and aids in proper functioning of the heart. A deficiency leads to an increased susceptibility to stress and other psychological disturbances, muscle pain, weakness, and cardiomyopathy. Doses of more than 400 mcg daily can result in loss of hair and fingernails, fatigue, irritability, nausea, and abdominal pain.

Best natural sources—Garlic, fish, shellfish, eggs, liver, red meat, nuts, especially Brazil nuts, and whole grains.

RDI—55 mcg daily for adults.

CAUTION

911!

Be careful when taking single ingredient mineral supplements. Minerals are designed to work together inside our bodies, and if we take too much of one it may result in a deficiency of another. Deficiencies compound because a lack of certain minerals makes it much more difficult to absorb other minerals. A balanced mineral supplement is your best bet because it contains the minerals your body needs in proper proportions.

Molybdenum—Serving as a catalyst for multiple enzyme reactions, molybdenum is also vital to the formation of blood, cartilage, and bone. Symptoms of deficiency may include irritability, intolerance for amino acids, and coma. There is no UL set for molybdenum; however, overdoses may lead to gout, hallucinations, and possibly seizures.

Best natural sources—Spinach, strawberries, milk, whole grains, legumes, liver, and dark green leafy vegetables.

RDI—75 mcg daily for adults.

Manganese—Magnesium is required for energy metabolism, wound healing, fertility, and assists in the formation of blood and bone. A deficiency may result in nausea and vomiting, nervous system disorders, or interference with metabolism and birth defects. There is no UL set for manganese; however, overdoses may result in episodes of psychosis.

Best natural sources—Whole grains, nuts, legumes, tea, cocoa powder, and oatmeal.

RDI—2 mg daily for adults.

Herbs—Ancient Remedies Rediscovered

Herbs may seem like the new kid on the block, but in reality, herbal medicine is thousands of years old. Practitioners of TCM, or Traditional Chinese Medicine, have been prescribing herbal concoctions for their patients for centuries, often with excellent results.

Still, a note of caution is in order. Just because a product is natural does not ensure that it is either safe or effective. People sometimes make the mistake of overdosing on herbs in the mistaken belief that herbal preparations are "safe" and cannot hurt them. Overdoses of herbs can be just as toxic and even as deadly as overdoses of any drug. The proliferation of herbs on the market coupled with conflicting claims of efficacy and the difficulty of obtaining solid clinical evidence to back claims makes getting reliable information about herbs very difficult.

Another problem is that the marketing of herbs is entirely unregulated. No agency oversees the claims made for various products or checks to make sure that pills are as potent as they claim or contain the amount of active ingredient claimed.

This is not to say that herbs cannot be very valuable to support health. Many of our most valuable medicines are derived from herbs. Just use common sense and do your homework. Make sure you follow dosage recommendations and that the herb you want to take doesn't conflict with any medications you are already taking. The best way to do that is to discuss the matter with your doctor.

There are literally thousands of herbs and herbal compounds that have been used with varying degrees of success practically from the dawn of recorded human history. To discuss each one even briefly here would produce a tome weighty enough to serve as the anchor on the USS *Enterprise*. Instead, we'll discuss the most popular herbs, the ones that have been much in the news of late.

- **St. John's wort**—Used for the treatment of mild to moderate depression, St. John's wort burst onto the scene a few years ago. Its historical uses include not only the treatment of anxiety, but also to soothe minor burns and to treat wounds and bruises.

- **Echinacea**—Stimulates the immune system and helps the body ward off opportunistic infections like colds and flu. Used in topical form, it also is an effective anti-inflammatory against skin conditions like psoriasis and eczema. It is particularly effective when used in combination with goldenseal.

- **Gingko biloba**—Gingko is a powerful antioxidant that enhances circulation, particularly to the brain, ears, eyes, heart, and limbs. Gingko improves memory and cognitive function and has been used with some success to treat senility and Alzheimer's disease and tinnitus or ringing in the ears.

- **Ginseng**—Used by Chinese herbalists for almost 5,000 years, it strengthens the immune system and builds resistance to the detrimental effects of stress. Because it increases stamina and vitality, it is frequently used in formulations to increase physical energy and reduce fatigue.

- **Saw palmetto**—Alleviates symptoms of enlarged prostate in men.

- **Red clover**—Helps relieve symptoms of menopause and offers a cardio-protective effect similar to that of estrogen in postmenopausal women.

- **Feverfew**—Anti-inflammatory used to treat migraines, reduce fever, reduce gassiness, and soothe indigestion.

- **Goldenseal**—Astringent and antibacterial, goldenseal is used to treat symptoms of cold and flu. It is particularly effective when used in combination with echinacea.

- **Valerian**—Mild sedative used to treat insomnia, nervous conditions, and to induce sleep.

- **Bilberry**—Enhances vision and is often used to treat night blindness. It also strengthens the walls of blood vessels and reduces inflammation.

All About Phytonutrients

You may be asking yourself, "What in the heck are phytonutrients?" Up until a decade ago, most scientists and nutrition researchers would have been scratching their heads right along with you.

The word *phyto* is actually derived from the Greek word for plant. Phytonutrients are pigments and flavonoids that occur in minute amounts in fruits and vegetables and yet give foods their characteristic colors, flavors, and odors. Until recently, it was thought that's all they were good for. But developing research is proving that phytonutrients play unique and essential roles in maintaining wellness.

Early research suggests that phytonutrients are potent antioxidants and free radical scavengers and that they strengthen the body's immune system, repair DNA damage cause by exposure to cigarette smoke and other toxic chemicals, detoxify carcinogens or cancer-causing substances, and most exciting of all, actually cause cancer cells to "commit suicide" through a process called *apoptosis*.

Wellness Words

Apoptosis is a biological regulatory mechanism through which damaged, old, or rogue cells kill themselves off in an orderly fashion, thereby maintaining a desirable state of homeostasis in the body. Also called PCD or programmed cell death.

Supplement companies are rushing to market their particular brand of phytonutrients, which are often very pricey, ranging from $50 or more for a one-month supply. The good news is that you can supply your body's requirements simply by including an adequate amount of raw food in your diet. If you have a sliced banana on your morning cereal, munch on carrots for snacks, eat tomatoes on your spinach salad at lunch, and enjoy a wedge of cantaloupe for dessert, you've consumed all the phytonutrients you need for the day. The only people who are deficient in phytonutrients are those who eat diets consisting almost entirely of junk food, fast food, and prepackaged meals.

The following phytonutrients have been identified by the Phytonutrients Laboratory at the U.S. Department of Agriculture:

♦ **Carotenoids**—Include the red, orange, and yellow pigments that give so many fruits and vegetables their appealing color. Alpha-carotene, beta-carotene, beta-cryptoxanthin, lutein, lycopene, and zeaxanthin have been identified so far. You might think that carotenoids are only present in red, orange, and yellow foods, but they are actually a significant component of many green leafy vegetables as well.

Benefits—Protects against heart disease, certain cancers and age-related muscular degeneration.

Best sources—Carrots, sweet potatoes, broccoli, kale, spinach, green leafy vegetables, turnips, pumpkins, citrus fruits, peaches, apricots, cantaloupes, tomatoes, watermelon, and others.

◆ **Polyphenols**—Divided into two categories: flavanoids and nonflavanoids. Flavanoids include flavones, flavanones, flavanols, isoflavones (also called phytoestrogens), catechins, anthocyanins, and quercetins. Nonflavanoids currently under study include ellagic acid and coumarin. In the scientific world, polyphenols are called secondary plant metabolites. They are not understood nearly as well as the carotenoids.

Benefits—Potent antioxidants and free radical scavengers, decreased risk of cardiovascular disease.

Best sources—Onions, apples, soybeans, citrus fruits, red grapes, grape juice, red wine, tea, strawberries, blueberries, raspberries, and cranberries.

◆ **Inositol phosphates**—Also called phytates, currently under study for the role they play in the prevention of certain cancers, including colon cancer.

Benefits—Regulates vital cellular functions and helps cancer prevention.

Best sources—Cereals and legumes and vegetable fiber like wheat, rice, and oat bran.

◆ **Lignans**—Also called phytoestrogens, may help prevent certain cancers, particularly breast cancer.

Benefits—Regulates glucose, regulates plasma lipids and blood pressure, cancer prevention, and acts as an anti-inflammatory.

Best sources—Seeds, particularly flaxseed, nuts, whole grains, and black and green tea.

◆ **Isothiocyanates**—Also called indoles, may help prevent gastrointestinal cancers and also lung, mouth, and throat cancers.

Benefits—Induces apoptosis in cancer cells and in carcinogenic substances that invade the body.

Best sources—Cruciferous vegetables, including broccoli, cabbage, kale, and cauliflower.

◆ **Phenols**—Also called cyclic compounds, may help prevent gastrointestinal cancers and also lung, mouth, and throat cancers.

Benefits—Cancer prevention, regulation of blood sugar, and alleviation of arthritis symptoms.

Best sources—Cruciferous vegetables, including broccoli and kale.

◆ **Saponins**—Used to make soap and provide the foamy head in root beer and other beverages.

Benefits—Lowers cholesterol, antifungal, antibacterial, prevention of colon cancer, increases the effectiveness of vaccines, and enhances immune system.

Best sources—Soybeans, peas, yucca, spinach, and oats.

◆ **Sulfides**—Also called thiols, a sulfur-containing class of compounds.

Benefits—Regulates serum cholesterol and triglycerides, prevention of heart disease, regulation of glucose, and acts as an immunity booster.

Best sources—Garlic, onions, and cruciferous vegetables.

◆ **Terpenes**—Also called indoles. In the plant world, these pungent chemicals are used to defend plants against attack by insects.

Benefits—Cancer protection.

Best sources—Peppermint, spearmint, lemon, lime, orange, and grapefruit.

The important thing to remember about nutrition and supplementation is that, despite all our knowledge and ongoing research, what we know about the subject is still relatively little. There may be whole classes of nutrients still out there waiting to be discovered. The use of minerals, herbs, and phytonutrients as supplements may be well advised for particular health situations and for a particular period of time. But do consult your doctor before taking any new supplement to make sure there are no medication conflicts or existing conditions that would suggest you should not take it. Finally, remember that the best way to healthy overall nutrition is to eat a balanced diet that contains some raw food every day.

The Least You Need to Know

◆ Minerals are just as essential to maintaining good health as vitamins.

◆ To ensure you get an adequate supply of minerals and phytonutrients, you should include some raw foods in your diet each day.

◆ If you do take mineral supplements, take a balanced formulation to ensure proper absorption.

◆ Herbs can be very beneficial in maintaining health, but overdoses can be toxic, and certain herbs may interfere with some prescription drugs.

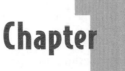

Chapter 12

Water, Water, Everywhere, and You Need Lots of Drops

In This Chapter

- What water does
- 48 ounces, 64 ounces—or more?
- Warning signs of dehydration
- Tap, bottled, or filtered

If food is the fuel that runs your body's engine, water is the oil, the antifreeze, and the brake and transmission fluid. It's what keeps everything running smoothly. In this chapter we'll tell you why it's so important to keep your body properly hydrated and give you a few tips to help make drinking enough water a bit more palatable.

So What's the Big Deal About Water?

When you talk about the importance of drinking enough water, some people are likely to be dismissive, as if it didn't matter whether or not they keep their bodies supplied with H_2O.

We need water, and we need it everyday. It's that simple. A person can survive 30 days or more without a bite of food, but take away his water and he'll be dead within a week.

Water serves many vital purposes in the human body. Getting an adequate amount is essential to keep our bodies functioning properly. Among its most important jobs, water …

- Regulates body temperature.
- Speeds digestion and elimination of waste.
- Lubricates and cushions joints.
- Moves nutrients throughout the body.
- Dissolves water-soluble vitamins so the body can utilize them.
- Is essential for all digestive, absorption, circulatory, and excretory functions.

Water is involved in every chemical and electrical reaction that goes on inside your body. Neglecting water intake can mean those reactions get derailed, with potentially deadly consequences.

The body loses about 10 cups of water per day on average, through the processes of urination, digestion, perspiration, and respiration. If you do not replenish your body's water stores on as regular basis, you can become dehydrated and put yourself at risk for several health problems. Dehydration has been implicated as a contributing factor in the development of kidney stones, muscle cramps, heat stroke, and even blood clots.

Can't I Get Some Water from My Food?

The good news is that it's easier to keep yourself hydrated than you may think. The food in a typical day's diet provides about four cups of water, meaning that you may drink as little as four additional eight-ounce cups of water per day and still meet your body's requirements. Here are some popular foods and their percentage of water content:

- Raw apples—85 percent
- Whole-wheat bread—35 percent
- Bananas—76 percent
- Broccoli—91 percent
- Broiled chicken—71 percent
- Peanut butter—trace amount
- Broiled veal—60 percent
- Watermelon—93 percent
- Smoked ham—54 percent

- Honey—15 percent
- Lettuce—96 percent
- Pecans—7 percent
- Sweet corn—74 percent
- Butter—20 percent
- Raw pears—82 percent
- Raw carrots—88 percent
- Grapes—82 percent
- American cheese—37 percent

Pure fats and oil have no water content whatsoever. Dried beans and grains generally have a water content of less than 10 percent, but that amount increases dramatically when the product is cooked in water or broth.

By selecting a balanced diet that includes plenty of fresh raw fruit and vegetables, you will be going a long way toward fulfilling your body's daily requirements for water, all without drinking a drop!

Trust Your Thirst

The human body is a wonder of design. We don't have to worry about when we need water because our bodies tell us by signaling thirst. Thirst is one of the body's most powerful regulatory mechanisms. First our lips start to feel dry, then our mouths, and finally our throats. Our natural response to these stimuli is to drink something.

When we respond to our thirst by drinking water, we switch off the thirst signal. However, sometimes we respond by eating instead of drinking. New research suggests an easy way to manage weight is to try drinking an eight-ounce glass of water when you think you're hungry. If you still feel hungry 20 minutes after drinking the water, then you probably really are hungry. But if you are actually thirsty instead of famished, drinking the water will make the feeling of hunger go away within 20 minutes.

From the Medicine Chest

Even if you don't pay much attention to the amount of water you take in, your body is right on top of it. When it loses 1 to 2 percent of its total volume of water through natural metabolic processes, your brain sends a thirst signal to special receptors in the back of your throat, prompting you to replenish your body's hydration by drinking water.

I Drink Coffee, I Drink Tea, So Why Do I Need Water?

Not everyone is thrilled with the idea of drinking plain old water. Some municipal tap water and even private well water can have an off taste or odor, and bottled water can be expensive. The same people who will happily guzzle a Gatorade or diet cola balk at the idea of swigging water all day long.

Do you really need to drink water? Can't you drink something else and get the same effect? This is another area where experts disagree. Some say only pure water can truly satisfy thirst and that water—not juice, not milk, not soda, coffee, or tea—is what your body needs to function properly. Others maintain any beverage will provide your body with some water.

But your body doesn't need just "some water." It needs quite a bit. If you want to truly enhance your wellness, drinking an adequate amount of water every single day is one of the best places to start.

Alcohol has such a powerful diuretic effect on the body that you end up with a net loss of water when you drink wine, beer, or cocktails. Some researchers have speculated that the intractable headaches that accompany a hangover may, in fact, be a sign of significant dehydration. If you're at a social event and know you'll be having several alcoholic beverages over the course of the evening, it's a good idea to intersperse those drinks with a tall glass of water to avoid problems with dehydration. Your head will thank you the next morning.

Caffeinated beverages like coffee, tea, and cola have a diuretic effect, which means they increase the amount of water your body excretes through your urine. Although some experts say caffeinated beverages can still provide your body with a net gain of water and drinking them is better than allowing yourself to become dehydrated, the truth is that they do not truly quench thirst. In fact, caffeine has just the opposite effect. It makes you feel thirstier. Second, these beverages add empty calories and very little nutritive value to your diet. Water has no calories and no added sugar and may also contain several valuable trace minerals, making it your best choice as a thirst quencher.

Are You Hungry or Thirsty?

People who have trouble losing weight even though they eat a balanced, moderate diet should look at their fluid intake. Alcoholic beverages are the third highest source of caloric intake in America, accounting for more than 5 percent of the total calories consumed each day. But that statistic doesn't convey the whole picture. Because many people do not drink alcoholic beverages at all, in reality the average adult drinker gets 10 percent of his daily calories from booze, while problem drinkers may get up to half their calories from alcohol.

CAUTION **911!**

Watch what you drink. Four of the top 10 grocery items sold in America are calorie-laden beverages, including soft drinks, juices, milk, and beer. According to the National Soft Drink Association, soda consumption in this country has almost tripled in the past 30 years. Make water your beverage of choice and you'll save all those empty calories. You could lose 20 pounds in a year simply by replacing one 16-ounce soda per day with a glass of water.

Why should you drink water? Because it's your body's perfect choice for hydration. Your body was designed to work with water, and no matter what anyone may tell you, it won't work as well if it doesn't get enough.

How Much Water Do I Really Need?

Like everything else that has to do with your health, experts can't agree on how much water you should be drinking. Their recommendations range from a low of four eight-ounce glasses (assuming you get an average of four cups daily in our food) to eight or more eight-ounce glasses daily at the minimum. Others say you should divide your weight by two to determine the number of ounces of water you should drink daily. For example, if you weigh 150 pounds, you should drink 75 ounces of water a day.

The American Dietetic Association recommends drinking 48 to 64 ounces daily and says that amount is adequate for most people.

Do You Get Enough Water?

Almost 60 percent of the respondents who took a recent online water intake survey said they drank from anywhere from three to eight 8-ounce glasses of water per day. But 3 percent of the respondents claimed that they hated water and never drink it. Since our bodies are approximately 65 to 75 percent water, with our brains topping out at 75 percent and our blood 83 percent water, the decision not to supply your body with one of it major components seems ill-informed at best.

The best way to determine how much water you need is to learn to recognize your own thirst. Start with the minimum recommended six eight-ounce glasses spread over the course of the day, and add water as your body asks for it.

Pay Attention to the Weather

If the weather is hot or you are going to be more active than usual, your body will require more water to stay properly hydrated. Be particularly careful to drink plenty of water if you are going to be outdoors for an extended period on a warm day. If you will be performing strenuous work like gardening or participating in an athletic event, you can get dehydrated very quickly if you don't maintain adequate water intake.

Athletes Have Special Requirements

People who exercise regularly do require additional water to make up for what they lose through perspiration. Experts say that for every thousand calories you expend in exercise, you need about four additional eight-ounce glasses of water to stay properly hydrated.

The sports drink Gatorade was introduced in 1965, launching an entire new industry. In addition to water and sugar, it contains the electrolytes sodium and potassium, which your body loses through perspiration during physical exertion. If you're an athlete in competition and you're worried about replacing electrolytes, an occasional sports drink might be a good choice.

Room Temperature or Cold?

Would you be surprised to learn there is even debate over the temperature of the water you drink? Some trainers swear by ice-cold water, saying that it cools you down in the middle of an intense workout. They also claim that warming the water to 98.6 degrees makes your body burn a few additional calories.

On the other side of the argument are doctors who say that ice-cold water can be a shock to the delicate lining of the stomach.

Water temperature boils down to a matter of personal preference. If you can't stand the thought of drinking water unless it is ice cold, then ice-cold water is what you should drink. If you prefer tepid or room temperature water, that's fine, too. The most important thing is that you just drink it, warm or cold, every single day, in sufficient quantity to keep your body properly hydrated.

When Not Drinking Can Be Deadly

It's easy to overlook the warning signs of dehydration, a potentially deadly condition that is your body's way of telling you that you are dangerously low on water reserves. Dehydration occurs when your body does not have enough water to carry on its normal metabolic activities. If you do not address it right away, you may develop heat exhaustion or even a heat stroke.

Learn these warning signs to protect yourself from dehydration:

Moderate dehydration, also known as heat exhaustion:

- Dry mouth and lips
- Thick tongue and thick saliva
- Extreme thirst
- Dizziness, weakness, and difficulty standing
- Cramping in the arms and legs
- Headache
- Dry, warm skin and flushed face
- Despite thirst, no desire or ability to drink
- Scant or very dark urine
- Feeling of malaise

Severe dehydration, also known as heat stroke:

- Loss of consciousness
- Low blood pressure
- Convulsions
- Heart failure
- Rapid, faint pulse
- Rapid breathing
- Severe muscle spasms in arms, legs, and back
- Wrinkled, loose skin

911!

Heat stroke is a medical emergency! Moderate dehydration can quickly become severe dehydration or heat stroke if not treated immediately. In severe dehydration, the feet and hands may begin to turn blue, a sign that the body is shutting down its extremities in a desperate effort to keep its central core cool. Unless a person who is severely dehydrated receives professional medical treatment immediately, death will soon follow.

Severe dehydration or heat stroke occurs when the body's temperature control mechanism stops working. Victims stop producing sweat, which is normally used to cool the body. The core temperature of the body can rise so high that it literally "cooks" the brain, resulting in severe brain damage, coma, or even death.

Raise your awareness to protect yourself from the dangers of dehydration. If you're working outside or participating in an outdoor event, make sure you get plenty of water throughout the day. Take frequent rest breaks. If you start feeling dizzy or light-headed, stop whatever you're doing immediately and seek medical attention.

What Kind of Water Should I Drink?

Now that you've determined to add drinking an adequate daily supply of water to your wellness agenda, you must decide what kind of water you will drink. From the tap, filtered, distilled, or bottled? Here are some tips to help you decide what's best for you.

Taps for Tap Water

The Environmental Protection Agency estimates that Americans drink more than one billion glasses of tap water per day. But tap water is not the best choice. Many municipal water supplies are so heavily chlorinated that drinking them could be detrimental to your health. The same chlorine that kills potentially dangerous water-borne bacteria and parasites is in itself toxic when ingested by humans or absorbed through the skin. It has been implicated in a variety of health problems, including suppression of the immune system, birth and developmental defects, infertility, neurological damage, and cancer, among others. The problem is so serious that many water-treatment facilities are currently investigating safer treatment methods, and some have already proposed eliminating chlorine treatment altogether.

Water from private wells may contain a variety of chemicals and pesticides that have leached into the groundwater. Even if the chemical is natural and beneficial, like sulfur, it can produce such a noxious taste and odor that it renders the water undrinkable.

Bottled Blues

Bottled water has grown into a $4 billion a year industry in the United States. Sales of certain categories, like Spring Water, are growing by as much as 25 percent a year.

One would like to be able to trust a bottle of water, but there have been several recent cases that proved bottled water is not always as pure as advertised. There was a famous case in Louisiana a few years back when a company was caught filling bottles of its famous "spring water" from a garden hose hooked up to the municipal water supply.

In addition, some bottled waters have been shown to contain bacterial contaminants and/ or synthetic chemicals that have leached from the plastic containers into the water. A few have tested positive for traces of deadly contaminants like arsenic.

Finally, bottled water is very expensive. Depending on your geographic location, it can cost as much as 5,000 times more per gallon than your local tap water.

No one can argue the convenience of bottled water, particularly for athletes and people on the move. You know it's found a permanent niche in the national consciousness when you can order it at a fast-food drive up, where it is the superior beverage of choice by far.

If you prefer bottled water, bottled spring water is the way to go. Spring water contains trace minerals like calcium and magnesium that support wellness, making it slightly alkaline and, therefore, ideal to meet your body's needs. Look for a brand from a reliable company.

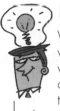

From the Medicine Chest

When buying bottled water, stay away from water packaged in soft, cloudy plastic bottles. This type of plastic leaches chemicals into whatever liquid is stored within. Instead, opt for hard, clear plastic bottles that do not leach chemicals.

It All Boils Down to This

For almost 50 years, health-conscious people thought drinking distilled water was the only way to go. Modern research suggests otherwise.

Distilled water is made by boiling water, evaporating it, and collecting the condensed vapor. It contains no minerals, and as a result, it behaves in what scientists have described as an "aggressive" manner inside your body, dissolving any chemical it comes into contact with. This can make your body slightly acidic, which is not desirable. People who drink distilled water exclusively may develop multiple mineral deficiencies.

Distilled water is the best choice if you want to detox or flush out your system but shouldn't be used for more than a couple of weeks. Choose spring water instead.

The Fuss over Filters

Despite what your local salesperson may tell you, you don't have to spend your child's inheritance on a whole-house water-treatment system to get good quality water. It can be as simple as buying a $25 pitcher equipped with a filter on the pouring spout or as complex as installing a $2,500 reverse osmosis system that treats every drop that comes into your house.

The argument for treating all your water is compelling. We do absorb chlorine through our skin, so many natural health practitioners now warn against bathing, showering, or swimming in chlorinated water. Chlorinated water is also very hard on clothing. That beautiful new sweater will fade and start to look old very quickly after a few cycles in the washer if your municipal water is heavily chlorinated. However, if you do not have a lot of money to invest, an under-the-sink or sink-top water filter to treat your family's drinking water is a good place to start. And don't forget to put a filter on the water line of your ice-maker as well.

Each filtration method has its particular strengths and weaknesses. Here are the most common:

- **Carbon block filter.** Water is filtered through the pores of a compacted carbon block. Relatively inexpensive, carbon filtration removes chlorine, particles, and most taste and odor problems without removing beneficial minerals. Because they do not require electricity to operate, carbon block filters are available to fit a variety of faucets, including sinks, tubs and showers, and outdoor spigots.

- **Reverse osmosis.** Water passes through a semi-permeable membrane that removes suspended particles, then goes to a holding tank where salt, nitrates, heavy metals, and other inorganic materials are removed. Reverse osmosis removes beneficial minerals but does not remove pesticides. Relatively slow and expensive, reverse osmosis can use three or more gallons of water to produce one gallon of drinkable water.

- **Granular activated carbon filter.** Removes chlorine, rust, and particles, but can grow bacteria unless treated with silver nitrate. Water can pass around the carbon granules without treatment, so this type of filter is frequently combined with micro-filters that also remove microscopic cysts that can cause illness. This treatment is less expensive than bottled water, but still more expensive per gallon than an under-the-sink unit.

- **Ultrafine ceramic cartridge.** The newest technology, these filters are impregnated with silver and remove bacteria, chlorine, parasites, cysts, organic chemicals, particles, and sediment and are ideal for use in portable filters where drinking water is suspect. The downside? They're expensive and not yet widely available in this country.

After comparing available models and features, choose the most effective filter you can afford. Home filtering is currently the best and most affordable way to provide safe drinking water for your family. No matter how much you decide to spend, remember it's an investment in your family's ongoing health and wellness.

The Least You Need to Know

- Adequate water intake is essential to your health.
- Experts recommend you drink a minimum of six to eight eight-ounce glasses of water per day.
- Thirst can sometimes masquerade as hunger.
- Severe dehydration is a medical emergency that can kill you very quickly.
- Using filters is the least expensive way to ensure the safety of your family's drinking water supply.

Part **3** The Second Pillar— Exercise—Get Up and Move

If you're the sort of person who might only get up from your recliner to exercise if someone was threatening to smash your remote control with a hammer, we've got some great ideas for you. If you truly want to incorporate wellness into your lifestyle, regular exercise is not optional—it's required.

Now, stop grimacing. Exercise can be fun and even a little addictive, especially when you start to see the results. The trick is to figure out your exercise style and then tailor a program that meshes with your needs and personal preferences.

In this part, we'll talk about the many benefits of regular exercise and provide an overview of various types of exercise programs, including aerobic and strength training. In a few short months of regular exercise, you will be seeing a whole new you.

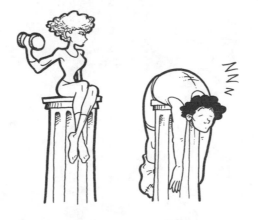

Why Do I Have to Exercise?

In This Chapter

- ◆ Exercise once was a part of daily living
- ◆ Every part of your body benefits from exercise.
- ◆ Five motivating reasons to exercise
- ◆ Exercise to feel better and have more energy

More than 100 years ago, very few people went out expressly to exercise, mostly because they didn't have to. Just living required a lot of hard physical labor from both men and women. Those were the days when people cleared the land, built their own homes, cared for their animals, and farmed. Travel of any distance required a horse and wagon, and they took care of both.

Women carried water from the well in heavy wooden buckets; they churned butter, scrubbed their floors on their hands and knees, and washed clothes by hand. Men chopped firewood, planted and harvested their crops, often working in their fields from dawn to dusk. Couples worked together to build their houses and barns and take care of their farms and animals. A family produced almost everything they needed with their own physical labor. A young couple in love might take a long walk, hand in hand, and talk about their future together, and that future probably involved working hard, together.

Those days are gone. Few individual farms are left. Just like the rest of us, you probably bought a home already built or maybe you live in an apartment. The land is already cleared, and the only animals you might have to take care of are a cat or a dog. You may jump onto the freeway to get to a job, and like millions of others, you will probably sit at a desk most of the day. Water? Just turn on the faucet. Heat or air conditioning? Just flip the switch on the wall. Floors dirty? Plug in the vacuum cleaner and, with a little effort, push it around. Young couples in love still hold hands, still talk about their future together, but they often do it seated in a fast-moving sports car.

I'm Out of Shape, and It's Jay Leno's Fault

It is no secret that many of us have gotten into the habit of stopping by a fast-food place after work to pick up something to reheat in the microwave. After kicking off your shoes, eating your food from a TV tray while you watch the news, it's so very easy to lay back in the recliner with the TV clicker in your hand. Later, you might heat up some popcorn or open a bag of pretzels or chips to eat as you watch the late night comedians.

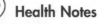 **Health Notes**

More than 60 percent of the adult population is not regularly active, and 25 percent of the adult population is not active at all.

You are not alone. According to A. C. Nielsen, the average American watches 3 hours and 46 minutes of TV daily.

I'm Soooo Tired

Just like the rest of us, you work hard all week. It might not be physical labor, but it is grueling and exhausting. You might head out the door on the weekend to play a pickup game with friends. Or you just might ride your bike a bit and then head to a local sports bar to drink beer and eat a burger.

Monday morning is a good time to complain about your hangover and how sore your muscles are after your weekend workout. Sound familiar?

Perhaps you're a person who doesn't spend a lot of time sitting around watching TV. Maybe you regularly do the chores around the house and you take care of the yard. You play with the kids, drive them to their soccer game or after-school activities, and take the dog for a walk. So you are thinking that when it comes to being active and getting exercise in your day-to-day activities you aren't doing too bad.

But perhaps you've begun to notice that your waistband is just a little bit tighter than it was last year at this time, and when you shopped for something new to wear you had to step it up one size. Size 6, if you ever wore it at all, is just something to wish for. Maybe you've begun to suspect that you aren't quite as fit as you want to believe you are.

If your clothes don't fit, your significant other seems to be looking at other people when the two of you are out together, or your doctor tells you that you need to do something about your blood pressure, your weight, or some of your other bad habits, and all you find yourself thinking is, "Nag, nag, nag." Well, maybe it is time for you to begin exercising, but you still need a compelling reason to start and haven't found one yet.

How does having a renewed zest for living, looking forward to plunging into the salt water of an ocean, walking in the woods, smelling the moist earth after a rain, looking forward to love making, and finding joy in your life sound?

Regular exercise, which will help you maintain optimum health and vitality, can do that for you.

Health Notes

By age 65 the average American will have spent nearly 9 years glued to the tube. Sixty-six percent watch television while eating dinner, and one in four will fall asleep with the TV on.

Physical Activity Is Essential for a Healthy Life

People are living longer despite a lack of exercise mostly because of medical discoveries such as antibiotics, vaccines, and better living conditions with sanitation and refrigeration. But those longer lives are often not healthy.

Nobody wants heart disease, diabetes, or colon cancer, but what does that mean for you?

The Centers for Disease Control reports that regular physical activity performed on most days of the week reduces the risk of developing or dying from the leading causes of illness and death in the United States, such as heart disease, diabetes, high blood pressure, and colon cancer.

Inactivity is one of the four major risk factors for heart disease. It is as important a risk factor as smoking, high cholesterol, and high blood pressure.

Exercise and Your Cardiovascular System

Exercise will lower your risk of developing coronary heart disease by 45 percent. Just like any other muscle, the heart can become stronger and larger and pump more blood. A healthy heart can pump more blood and sustain that work longer with less strain. While moderate dietary changes improve cholesterol levels, the lowered coronary artery risk occurs only if your regime includes some aerobic exercise. Exercise will lower your risk of developing high blood pressure or hypertension by 35 percent. Studies have indicated that high-intensity exercise does not lower blood pressure as effectively as moderate-intensity exercise. Although no one with hypertension should start an exercise program without consulting their physician, one study showed that moderate exercise controlled hypertension well enough that more than half of the people enrolled in it, under the supervision of their doctor, were able to discontinue their medication. Tai chi, the ancient Chinese discipline that involves slow, deliberate movement and is often performed in beautiful, tranquil settings such as green spaces, along the beach, or in public parks, lowers blood pressure almost as well as moderate-intensity aerobic exercise, such as jogging several miles a day.

By exercising, you will also increase your oxygen consumption by 20 percent. Increased oxygen consumption means that the heart, which is a muscle, is able to increase the volume of blood it pumps. The capacity of the blood to carry oxygen to all the cells in the body is increased. The skeletal muscle and the ability of that muscle to utilize the oxygen supplied to it is increased, making thinking, working, and breathing all easier.

Exercise can decrease pain from clogged arteries in the legs. It will make it possible for people who have intermittent claudication to triple the amount of time they can walk before they begin to feel pain.

Exercise and Your Muscles, Bones, and Joints

Exercise will increase flexibility, muscle strength, and endurance. Increased flexibility will make moving a lot easier. As one example, many people find they are no longer able to turn their heads to look over their shoulders, making driving dangerous. Muscle strength and endurance will make it easier to do your household chores, complete a workout, enjoy sex, go grocery shopping, and join others in volunteer activities such as fund-raising walkathons, or something even more simple, just make it possible to walk in the neighborhood with a friend. It will reduce pain and stiffness. People with osteoarthritis should avoid high-impact sports such as jogging and tennis.

There are types of exercise that are best for people with pain and stiffness: range of motion strength training, resistance training, and aerobics. Strength training includes isometric exercises, which means pushing or pulling against resistance and stretching without unduly stressing the joints. Low-impact aerobics will assist in stabilizing and supporting the joints and can even reduce inflammation in some of them. Research indicates that osteoarthritis sufferers often find that weakness in leg muscles is the cause of their osteoarthritis and pain. Strengthen those leg muscles and you might be able to say bye-bye to pain. Both swimming or water aerobics are excellent exercise choices for people with pain and stiffness, and cycling and walking are good beneficial choices as well.

Adding weight-bearing exercise will increase bone density by as much as 8 percent a year. Weight-bearing exercise encourages the body to compensate for the added stress. High-impact weight-bearing exercises are very protective of bone density for premenopausal women, but they increase the risk for osteoporotic fractures in the elderly, who would benefit more from regular and brisk walks. Even moderate exercise as little as one hour per week will assist in reducing the risk of fractures. Exercises that increase the focus on balance and strength, such as yoga, decrease the risk of falling, one of the potential problems that contribute to fractures in older women.

Exercise will improve symptoms for those who suffer from lower back pain. Eighty percent of all adults have experienced lower back pain sometime during their lifetime. Exercises that focus on flexibility and strengthening the abdominal muscles will help prevent recurring back problems. The best exercises are yoga, swimming, walking, and cross-country skiing. Partial sit-ups that maintain the back's normal curve can prevent lower back stress, but the classic full sit-up should be avoided.

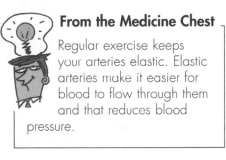

From the Medicine Chest

Regular exercise keeps your arteries elastic. Elastic arteries make it easier for blood to flow through them and that reduces blood pressure.

Exercise and Obesity

Exercise will burn calories and help fight obesity. If caloric intake remains the same, regular workouts will bring weight loss. It takes walking 35 miles to reduce 1 pound of body fat. A recent study reported that for the obese, a beginning daily session of exercise of only 10 minutes was helpful in assisting them to commit and adhere to a more vigorous exercise program. Swimming is less effective for weight loss than some other forms of exercise, such as walking or cycling, but for some people, swimming, with its factor of added buoyancy, may be an appropriate place to begin.

Exercise and Cancer

Exercise will reduce the risk for prostate, colon, and possibly breast cancer. There have been a number of studies that indicate that regular, moderate exercise reduces the risk of colon cancer and will help reduce the risk for prostate cancer. In the case of breast cancer, the benefits will depend on the woman's menstrual status and her estrogen levels.

From the Medicine Chest

If you are just beginning to exercise, pay attention to your breathing. When you can no longer do whatever it is, but have to suck the air in through your mouth, it is time to slow down. Nose breathing only will tell you when you can move up the intensity, the length of time, or the distance.

Exercise and Other Illnesses

Working out will reduce the risk for intestinal disorders such as ulcers, irritable bowel syndrome, indigestion, and diverticulosis. Exercise that strengthens the abdominal and pelvic muscles will combat constipation that will, in turn, reduce the risk of intestinal disorders.

Aerobic exercise reduces the risk of developing noninsulin-dependent diabetes, increases sensitivity to insulin, lowers blood pressure, improves cholesterol levels, and decreases body fat. Individuals who are insulin-dependent or who have diabetic complications need to discuss any exercise regime with their doctor before they begin.

Regular exercise also improves mobility and reverse muscle atrophy for people with multiple sclerosis, Parkinson's disease, and Alzheimer's. Specialized exercise programs will improve mobility, decrease spasticity, and provide improved psychological health. Exercise machines, pool exercises, and walking are particularly helpful. In addition, exercise will reduce the annual days lost to illness by five. Although there are no studies that indicate exercise improves the health of the immune system, a reduction in sick days taken each year was evident in studies of employees who participated in exercise programs as compared to those who did not.

Exercise, Sleep, and Mood

Exercise will increase feelings of well-being. Periods of intense training or longer aerobic workouts can raise levels of important brain chemicals such as the endorphins, which have been well documented to produce what is known as the *runner's high*. Teenagers actively engaged in sports have an increased sense of self-esteem. The more vigorously they participated in their chosen sport, the better their emotional well-being.

Working out can improve mental vigor, reaction time, acuity, math skills, creativity, and imagination. Both aerobic and nonaerobic workouts contribute to increased mental vitality. In one study, older individuals who exercised responded to mental challenges as quickly and as well as some younger adults. In a study of individuals who began a running program, they consistently scored higher on intellectual tests and showed significant improvement in memory and other mental skills, known as cognitive functioning. Maintaining a healthy flow of blood and oxygen appears to protect the brain.

Exercise will combat stress, anxiety, and sleeplessness. The side effects of the use of sedative hypnotic medications include confusion, falls, extended drowsiness, agitation, and problematic interactions with other medications. After 16 weeks in a moderate-intensity exercise program, participants were able to fall asleep about 15 minutes earlier and sleep about 45 minutes longer each night—a much better, healthier way to resolve sleep problems. Exercise has been shown to dramatically support a return to proper sleep cycles.

Working out has been shown to improve mood in people with clinical depression as effectively as some common forms of psychotherapy. Those who participated in a study in which they exercised with others, whether in a gym setting or walking on a track, improved more rapidly with the inclusion of the socialization factor than those who exercised alone.

Exercise and Pregnancy

Pregnant women may improve their chance for a timely delivery by exercising. All pregnant women should avoid high-impact, jarring exercises such as aerobic classes and step classes, which can weaken the muscles of the pelvic floor that support the uterus. Walking is an excellent exercise for pregnant women, and to strengthen the pelvic muscles in preparation for delivery, women can perform Kegel exercises a number of times a day. Kegel exercises involve repeatedly contracting the muscles around the vagina and the urethra for three seconds. This is one of those exercises you can do while standing in line at the check-out counter—no one is aware that you are exercising.

Health Notes

Although your brain is only 2 percent of your body's mass, it requires 25 percent of your blood supply.

Exercise and Sex

Fitness will improve your sex life. A toned and fit body is definitely sexy. Increased brain chemicals make sex more pleasurable. Increased flexibility and stamina will support and promote vigorous sexual performance. Exercise raises levels of important brain chemicals such as endorphins, adrenaline, serotonin, and dopamine—all of which produce feelings of pleasure. Endorphins are the brain's painkiller and are three times more powerful than morphine. Adrenaline provides a sense of being awake and alert. Serotonin helps maintain a feeling of happiness. Dopamine produces feelings of satisfaction, often reducing the desire to overeat.

In fact, there isn't even one part of your body, from the top of your head to the bottoms of your feet, that won't benefit from some exercise!

Get Moving

If you have been inactive for a while, it is probably a good idea to start with some less vigorous activities, such as walking or swimming at a comfortable pace. By starting out slowly, you can become fit without straining yourself. Once you begin to feel that you are in better shape, you can move on to a longer workout period and one that is more demanding.

Studies show that it is never too late to start exercising and even small improvement in physical fitness can significantly lower the risk of dying.

There are two types of exercise: aerobic and anaerobic (resistance training). Both are important to being healthy and fit.

Aerobic Exercise

Aerobic exercise is long in duration but low in intensity. It elevates the heart rate and breathing for a sustained period of time. It improves the efficiency of your heart and lungs, aids in controlling weight, and increases muscle and joint flexibility. Aerobic exercise is the kind of exercise most people should begin with, and it should leave you feeling like you have worked, that your heart rate was increased, and that your breathing was stimulated.

Regular aerobic exercise—brisk walking, jogging, swimming, biking, aerobic dance, and racquet sports—are the best forms of exercise for cardiac strengthening and for lowering LDL and raising HDL cholesterol levels.

Anaerobic Exercise

Anaerobic exercise is short in duration but emphasizes building muscle rather than burning oxygen. It strengthens the major muscle groups and reduces the stress of impact forces, lessening the risk of exercise-related injuries. Strength helps everyone perform all the daily tasks of living with greater ease. Those chores that have often left you huffing and puffing, such as climbing stairs, lifting boxes, house cleaning, and lawn care, become so much easier to do once you start exercising that you will no longer wish you had someone strong enough to do them for you.

Resistance training is important because it is the only form of exercise that will slow and even reverse the decline in muscle mass, bone density, and strength. Some common examples are football, push-ups, pull-ups, weight lifting, or any load-bearing activity.

Pick Five

Make a list of five ways you would benefit from getting regular exercise. It shouldn't take much thought to see areas of your life where being more flexible, for example, would increase your joy in living.

Write them in a proactive form; in other words, write: "I, (your name), will (ride my bike, take a yoga class, learn tai chi) because it will increase my flexibility, making it possible for me to bend over and pick up Fluffy so I can pet and cuddle her."

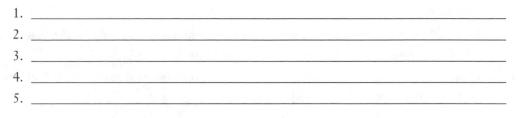

1. _____

2. _____

3. _____

4. _____

5. _____

By writing your personal exercise benefits in your own handwriting, you activate an area of your brain involved in mental alertness. That will help you focus on the benefits you will get from them and make these changes a reality for you.

The Least You Need to Know

- ◆ Years ago people worked so hard they didn't need additional exercise programs.
- ◆ The many benefits of exercise throughout your body are here for you to see.
- ◆ List five benefits you can use to help you focus on exercising.
- ◆ The ultimate benefit is that you will not only look younger, you will feel better.

Chapter 14

Fighting the Slide—How Exercise Keeps You Young

In This Chapter

- ◆ Trying to look and feel younger
- ◆ The multibillion-dollar youth industry
- ◆ Avoid the disabilities associated with aging and reverse the aging process
- ◆ How to *really* look and feel younger

Everybody wants to look younger. Everybody. Anyone who says that it isn't so is probably telling a big ol' fib.

When someone says, "Oh, you look so young," most of us reply with a smile and a generous "Thank you!" Of course you're flattered, pleased, and secretly happy that the person talking hasn't noticed your latest gray hair, the deepening of the crows' feet around your eyes, and that little bit of extra fat that recently appeared on your butt, thighs, or waist. Because, admit it, you are quite aware of them.

Very few people want to tell the truth about their age. Well, maybe your neighbor is happy to show you the photos of her great-great-grandchildren, but she is the exception.

Reversing the Aging Process

Color your hair; whiten your teeth; inject Botox into your wrinkles; get plucked, tweaked, and waxed; and then slather on the latest cream, ointment, or unguent with magic anti-aging ingredients. Get a tattoo, get your tattoo removed, and pierce your eyebrow and your navel. Make an appointment for breast implants, a face-lift, a hair transplant, and/or liposuction. Are these things the answer to the search for how to look younger, or do they just cost a lot of money—sometimes thousands—while the majority of them are only temporary and only cosmetic improvements?

It would be wonderful if just taking the cosmetic steps of doing everything you can to look younger would also make you feel younger. Unfortunately, while you might experience a little shopper's high, there is a let down to follow because they either don't do what you expect them to do, or they don't last.

The truth is, there really is a fountain of youth. Although Ponce de Leone looked for it in vain, it is now well documented that there is a method to not only feel younger, healthier, and more vibrant, but also look years younger at the same time—the "altar of exercise."

In several university studies, people who dedicated themselves to a variety of exercise regimes that included strength training not only looked younger, but also drastically reduced their measurable results on biological markers for aging such as reflexes, body fat composition, strength, coordination, lung function, and skin elasticity—sometimes reducing their biological ages as much as 15 to 20 years.

Results at the University of Texas Medical Branch in Galveston reported that the test individuals who were regularly physically active were slowing down the aging process and preventing chronic conditions from developing. They were *actually growing younger*, no matter what their birth certificates said.

The Multibillion-Dollar Industry

Looking for the appearance of youth has become a multibillion-dollar industry. There are dozens of perfect, slender, beautiful, young people staring back at you from the covers of the magazines that fill the racks at the grocery store checkout. These magazines are crammed with articles about how to look better in 15 minutes, supported with photos of these ravishingly lovely individuals. These are fantasy people, airbrushed to perfection, and the articles that accompany these photos will tell you the details of the latest diet and the latest must-have item you need to buy. And it will make your life miserable if you try the impossible—to look and be like them.

It is frightening to even think about movies and television, an unreal world where anyone much over 30 gets to play the mom or the dad in a sitcom. The music video channels can let you know 24 hours a day that there aren't any old people anywhere in the world. A recent article about Hollywood reported that many of the very fancy stores on Rodeo Drive only carry expensive women's clothing in sizes 0 to 6.

What are the rest of us, those approaching 25 or (yikes!) 30 and those who might be just a little tiny bit older than 30 or heavier than a size 6, to do?

Lookin' Good

In a recent study men and women of various ages were asked to have a brief conversation with a number of strangers in a mall and then decide whether or not they would consider each particular stranger *young* or *old*.

Many of these people measured the strangers against family members. Although they said they loved their older relatives, they definitely did not want to look like them or act like them as they themselves got older. The following table lists some of the things they observed in the strangers that influenced their decision.

Young	Old
Good posture	Stooped posture
Moist, dewy skin	Dry, withered skin
Nice hands	Age spots on hands
Ability to move	Doddering
Flexible	Stiff
Alert	Unconscious
Vital	Dried up
Mentally sharp	Forgetful
Unwrinkled	Prune-faced
Toned	Flabby
Full of life	Slow
Lively	Dull
Strong	Weak
Energetic	Weary
Firm	Saggy
Intelligent	Stupid
Rested	Tired
Vivacious	Lethargic

Health Notes

All the cells in your body are constantly renewing themselves. Ninety-eight percent of all your cells renew in one year. Every three months your skeleton is renewed. Every six weeks your liver renews itself. Every month your skin cells are new. Every five days your stomach has a new lining.

Of course, not every item on the list was observed in every stranger, but the picture the list paints is certainly not a pretty image of how another person should behave and look to give the impression of looking and being *old*.

Biological Markers

Researchers at Tufts University's Human Nutrition Research Center have listed 10 indicators or biomarkers that can be measured to determine your biological age, an age that can be quite different from your chronological age.

- Loss of lean muscle mass
- Loss of strength
- Basal metabolic rate
- Ratio of body fat to muscle
- Aerobic capacity
- Blood-sugar tolerance
- Cholesterol/HDL ratio
- Blood pressure
- Bone density
- Internal temperature regulation

Some of these biomarkers require special tests and evaluation to prepare a report result for any individual, such as bone density and aerobic capacity, but your physician, who can assess your blood pressure and perform a simple blood test to check your cholesterol and your blood glucose levels, can evaluate the rest.

Change Those Biomarkers

What one thing will have a tremendous impact on these biomarkers and make a difference in how young you look and feel? That one thing is? Right. You guessed it. *Exercise*.

Repeating over and over to yourself as you are drifting off to sleep, "Size 6. Size 6. Size 6," just won't do it. For the guys, sticking a poster of some wrestling hunk on your wall to gaze at once in a while won't make it happen for you, either. You are going to have to move if you want those images you dream about for yourself to become a reality.

♦ **1. and 2. Those first two biomarkers of biological aging, loss of lean muscle mass and strength, are important factors in the aged appearance of weakness that comes with them,** such as the inability to get up out of a chair, climb a flight of stairs, or lift a bag of groceries into the trunk of your car, and can all be reversed with some resistance training exercise. As your lean muscle mass and strength increase, you will find that you have increased energy. You'll also trim and tighten your entire body while controlling your weight and increasing your flexibility. You will look younger, feel better, easily handle that bag of groceries, glide to your feet without assistance after sitting a while—and that previously dreaded flight of stairs will be a snap.

♦ **3. Basal metabolic rate.** Your basal metabolic rate is a measurement of the amount of energy your body requires every day to perform its most basic functions like breathing, digesting your food, and circulating the blood throughout your body. This is a measurement of the amount of energy you would require if you really only did the couch potato thing all day long and never moved a muscle. Every 10 years your metabolic rate decreases, which means your body burns 100 less calories each day. Exercise helps your metabolism become more efficient, holding back that slide into the metabolic rate decrease that accompanies aging. You will burn more calories, even at rest. A well-conditioned body enables you to fall asleep faster, a fit body is ready to get moving more rapidly in the morning, and a more efficient metabolism improves the quality of your rest. You will not only look and feel more rested and refreshed when you get up in the morning, you'll be ready and raring to get going.

♦ **4. Ratio of body fat to muscle.** This simple measurement is done with a small pair of caliper on your upper arm. Or it can be done in an immersion tank that measures the floatability of fat. Any exercise, any at all, will alter the ratio of body fat to muscle. Any time spent exercising is worthwhile, even if you can only do it in brief spurts. That could mean parking your car at the farthest spot in the parking lot, taking the stairs instead of the elevator, or marching in place while you watch TV, if that is all the time you can find to devote to it. In just a few weeks of exercising, your skin all over your body will look and feel smoother, younger, and more supple, because you will be decreasing fatty tissue and increasing mass, and, therefore, stretching your skin tighter. This will be particularly noticeable on your shoulders and upper arms, and if you dread being seen in a bathing suit, the flesh around your buttocks and thighs will look tighter and firmer, too. You will feel stronger, look stronger, and be able to perform a lot more of the youthful things that more muscle makes possible.

> ### Health Notes
>
> A 22-week walking program for people in their 70s reversed 22 years of declining lung capacity.
>
> A 12-week weight resistance program more than doubled the leg muscle strength of participating women.
>
> A 12-month resistance training increased muscle strength of both participating men and women by 30 to 100 percent in the first 3 months.
>
> A walking program also improved the ability of the participants to climb stairs, stoop, crouch, kneel, and carry objects.
>
> In a 2-year study of healthy but inactive people over age 60, 13 percent developed new heart problems. In a parallel study of healthy and active people, only 2 percent developed similar problems.

◆ **5. Aerobic capacity.** This measures the ability of your muscles to absorb oxygen for use as fuel. This test is performed on a treadmill with specialized equipment that measures oxygen uptake. Most of us don't need a test; you know when you are panting for breath and just how long it takes you to reach that point. Aerobic capacity is fundamental to your ability to sustain exercise for any period of time. The higher your aerobic capacity, the greater your ability to perform everyday tasks with less fatigue, more energy, and the ability to increase your exercise performance. Aerobic capacity will decrease 10 percent each decade unless you take action to stop this from happening. That action, of course, is aerobic exercise of some sort. As you increase your heart rate you are replenishing the oxygen in your entire circulatory system, oxygenating your skin, brightening your complexion, putting a sparkle in your eyes, and renewing blood cells that will stimulate and nourish your hair and nails.

From the Medicine Chest

A sedentary 25-year-old can have less aerobic capacity than an active 50-year-old.

◆ **6. Blood sugar tolerance.** If your doctor suspects you might be at risk for developing diabetes, there are several tests he can prescribe to measure your blood glucose. The major chronic and debilitating illnesses that come with diabetes are serious: poor blood flow to your extremities with the resultant nerve damage and loss of feeling or painful burning feet. It is the main cause of blindness, the main cause of kidney failure, and a contributing factor to gum infections, which, if untreated, can result in the loss of your teeth. Exercise takes some of the glucose out of the blood to use for energy during and after exercise, automatically lowering blood glucose levels, which helps prevent these major illnesses. Preserving those physical functions necessary to a dynamic lifestyle and youthful appearance cannot be overemphasized. The prevention of chronic and serious illnesses is a large part of feeling healthy, resilient, and youthful.

◆ **7. Cholesterol/HDL ratio.** A blood test will give you these results. When there is too much cholesterol (a fatty substance) in your blood, it builds up on the walls of your arteries. Over time, this buildup causes hardening of the arteries so that they become narrowed and blood flow is blocked to the heart. Although high cholesterol is not visible, it contributes to the heart conditions that make ease of movement, endurance, and the ability to perform the tasks of daily living difficult. Exercise widens and strengthens your arteries, improving the flow of blood to the heart.

◆ **8. Blood pressure.** Your blood pressure is a measurement of the pressure the blood circulating in your body exerts against the walls of your arteries. Exercise, of course, will assist you to manage stress, reduce obesity, and increase the ability of your heart to pump blood more efficiently. Keeping your blood pressure under control will help you avoid heart disease, kidney disease, and stroke, all factors that contribute to chronic conditions, rapid aging, and the risk of death.

Wellness Words

The word **systole** means contraction. It is used to describe the heart when its rhythm forces the blood out. The word **diastole** means the opposite, the dilation of the heart, during which time it fills with blood.

◆ **9. Bone density.** Bone density is a measurement taken with specialized equipment that measures the weight of your skeleton overall or in specific regions. Important measurements are in the spine, hips, and arms, because these are the areas most likely to fracture when bone mass is low. This test isn't necessary, unless your physician orders it, but anyone can increase her bone density by resistance training, which includes walking (in which resistance comes from the legs pressing against the walking surface). Keeping your bones strong is particularly important for postmenopausal women to prevent bone demineralization, which contributes to a stooped posture, the "Dowager's hump" on the back of the neck, but most important, it will help to avoid the fractures of osteoporosis.

◆ **10. Internal temperature regulation.** The ability to regulate your temperature decreases with inactivity and age. Unless you increase your ability to remove body heat, you could suffer heat stroke. A well-conditioned athlete can run without feeling out of breath or breaking into a sweat. However, sweating will help your body

Health Notes

The average person loses seven pounds of muscle mass per decade once they have reached adulthood.

remove toxins as you increase your aerobic abilities. Sleeping well, waking up with glowing skin, and feeling focused and in balance are all benefits that can come with increasing your body's ability to regulate internal temperatures.

Here's Looking at You, Stranger

If you will recall the list of things the study group reported gave the appearance of not only looking old, but of being old, you won't find any mention of biological markers. A number of these markers, such as basal metabolic rate, blood pressure, or internal temperature regulation, are not readily visible, although lack of lean muscle mass, with flabby bellies, weak, spindly arms and legs, and body fat are easily noticeable. All the biological markers will respond positively to exercise because it is inactivity that results in a rapid rate of muscle atrophy, limited endurance, and the loss of flexibility and balance.

If you will exercise, those descriptive adjectives—stooped, doddering, slow, weak, and saggy—can't be applied to your healthier body and your youthful appearance. As your appearance, mental functioning, and mood improve, people will find you more fun to be with, more interesting, and maybe a potential love connection. With exercise you *can* reverse the aging process. So what about some of the other things on the list such as age spots and wrinkles?

Keeping Your Skin Young

Skin is the largest organ of the body, and yes, it is an organ. It has a number of tasks to perform besides keeping all of your insides inside. Among other things, it protects underlying tissues, helps control body temperature, stores some chemicals, and synthesizes several important compounds, like vitamin D. Age spots are sun damage. They can be removed by laser treatments and avoided by regularly using a sunscreen. Wrinkles, too, are the result of sun exposure, but some of them are the inevitable result of normal aging. Splotchy skin is often the result of stress that increases the production of several skin-damaging hormones. Better sleep cycles will help you not only feel better, but look more rested and younger.

Skin needs two basic things to look healthy: oxygen and hydration. So drink your water and indulge in some heavy breathing.

Maintaining Vitality Brain to Toe

Stupid, forgetful, and dull are adjectives often used to describe someone who appears to be getting mentally lazy. Remember: You have to pump blood up to your brain to keep it working properly. Add some mental exercise such as puzzles or board games like chess and Scrabble or play a musical instrument. Take up a hobby or learn to do something new. All these things will help keep your mind and memory tuned up.

With exercise strengthening your muscles, heart, and bones, it boosts your metabolism so you can eat an extra 300 calories a day and not gain any weight. It reduces negative moods because of the release of endorphins. Your sex life will be improved because of an increased blood supply to your pelvis. Men find that they have increased levels of testosterone and a higher body temperature—a physical reaction connected to arousal. Cancer rates are lower because exercise may boost the immune system's ability to detect and kill cancer cells. Stretching improves your range of motion, reduces pain, and helps maintain joint mobility so you appear toned, energetic, and full of life and vitality. If you want to be out there dancing with the younger crowd, movin' and groovin', it is time to get busy and exercise.

Visible or not, every single one of these attributes can be affected positively by exercise.

So spend your money on expensive creams and get a tummy tuck if that is what you want to do. These cosmetic changes may make you look a little better on the outside, but they won't improve your health. Look younger, feel younger, and enjoy having more energy, vigor, and vitality. All these beneficial, healthy, and youthful changes can be done with just one little item, one inexpensive item, one lifestyle change that researchers at the University of Texas Medical Branch in Galveston say will actually reverse the aging process itself—exercise.

The Least You Need to Know

- Everybody wants to look younger, be healthier, and feel younger.
- The multibillion-dollar beauty industry will make you unhappy with the way you look and provide you with cosmetic fixes that are no more than that.
- Many of the disabilities associated with being old can be avoided—and you may even reverse the aging process.
- Use it or lose it! If you really want to look healthy, feel healthy, and be healthy, you must exercise.

Chapter 15

Overcoming Inertia—No, Clicking Your Remote Is NOT Exercise

In This Chapter

- ◆ The hardest part is getting started
- ◆ The next hardest part is staying active
- ◆ Some theories about exercise
- ◆ Getting there and staying there

Some wise old guy, maybe it was Socrates or Confucius, said something like, "Every journey begins with just one step." Trite as that may seem right now, it is true, and when it comes to getting started with exercising, that wise old guy was right.

It doesn't matter what kind of shape you are in: if you already weigh 350 pounds and think it's hopeless, if you used to be in tip-top form and just slacked off, if you had an injury that put you out of commission for a while, if you've had a project at work that kept you working late, if by the time you put the kids to bed you're exhausted, or if you've been sitting on your duff for the last 10 years.

Your excuse really doesn't matter. What does matter is whatever it is that will get you going and keep you working out. If you've never exercised or you haven't been exercising for a while and you need something to get you started, that first step is the beginning for everyone no matter who they are or what shape they are in. You have to take that first step.

The Famous Midnight "Resolution"

The Babylonians celebrated New Year's Day more than 4,000 years ago as part of their spring ceremonies when they planted their crops. New Year's for them took place in March. They used that occasion to look over the happenings of the past year and to look forward to their expectations for the coming year.

For centuries people have taken the new year as an occasion to reflect on wanted or needed changes for the coming year. Almost everyone makes New Year's resolutions, and almost everyone gives up on them within the first month or so. Many people make resolutions *knowing* they are going to abandon them very shortly; some are dumped as early as the very next day.

A few months into the new year, many people no longer even remember what their resolutions were. They weren't really making promises to themselves; they were simply hoping that saying them would magically make them happen.

Resolving to make a change doesn't have to take place only at New Year's. You can see something about your behavior you're unhappy with and resolve to make changes any day. Keeping that resolve is another story.

Any time you find you are muttering to yourself things like, "I gotta get more exercise," "I gotta stop smoking," or "I gotta go to church," you are making a promise, a resolution. That resolution or promise is almost always to yourself, because you realize that what you are doing is not good and you would really like to change. A resolution with a "gotta" is only a half-baked promise of change.

Researchers have compiled a list of the most frequently pledged resolutions. You can be sure there is something on that list you have promised yourself you will either do—or stop doing.

The following are the most frequently made resolutions:

- ◆ Exercise more.
- ◆ Lose weight.
- ◆ Get in shape.
- ◆ Get a new job.
- ◆ Smile more.

◆ Quit smoking.

◆ Quit drinking.

◆ Get a life.

◆ Eat better.

◆ Save more money.

◆ Relax more.

◆ Get more sleep.

◆ Get organized.

◆ Go to church.

◆ Drop a dress size.

From the Medicine Chest

Researchers at the University of Washington found that 63 percent of the people they questioned remained at least semi-faithful to their number-one resolution for less than the first two months. And that number-one resolution: Exercise more. Hope you noticed that *semi*-faithful, because we all know what that means.

Researchers also found that while the majority vowed to do something they thought would be beneficial, they gave the implementation of their resolutions very little thought. Most thought they *ought* to do these things, but gave very little consideration about the *how* when they declared their New Year's resolutions.

The world is filled with backsliders, and you certainly don't want to be one of them. A resolution or a promise needs to be a commitment to yourself to do something. Because exercise is our topic here, your resolution might be to begin exercising or to exercise more. Such a promise made to yourself, made as a whim or made at the last minute, is a guaranteed formula for failure.

Making That First Step

You've been thinking that you really need to start exercising; you already know at least a dozen reasons why you should. You've resolved to begin several different times, but that resolve seemed somehow to get lost in all the other things you need to do. You also know another dozen reasons why it would be good for you, but you just can't seem to get started.

You have one excuse after another: "The weather is too bad. I don't have the right clothes. I don't have the right shoes, I'd go for a walk but I don't have anyone to walk with. If I go to the gym people will laugh at me. The gym isn't easy to get to. I hate exercise. Joining a gym is too expensive."

From the Medicine Chest

◆ Eliminate the negative.

◆ Learn from your mistakes and move on.

◆ Realize what is unimportant so you can focus on what is.

◆ Keep reinforcing positive achievement.

◆ Use achievement, no matter how small, to build your self-confidence.

Once you figure out some answers that will blow these excuses away, you can get creative with a whole new set of obstacles: "I didn't sleep well last night and I don't feel very good. I think I'm coming down with a cold. I don't want to get all sweaty and mess up my hair. I have people coming over and I have to fix something for dinner."

Sound familiar?

Excuses, Excuses

You've got a pretty good list of excuses; they're actually pretty creative. Let's write down at least five of them.

1. _____
2. _____
3. _____
4. _____
5. _____

All right, we've admired your creativity. Now, let's rewrite that list and change your excuse into a reason. The difference between an excuse and a reason is that the reason will have a rational motive that supports that conclusion.

An example:

Excuse: I don't have the right shoes.

Reason: I don't have the right shoes, and I can't afford to buy them right now.

Very good. An excuse and a reason to justify it.

Now, let's rewrite the list one more time and this time, add a *because* and a *but* to the end of that reason.

Example: I don't have the right shoes, and I can't afford to buy them right now *because* I really want those expensive pro-athlete ones, *but* I could get a cheaper, generic pair from the discount store.

1. _____
2. _____
3. _____
4. _____
5. _____

When you write it like this, you not only have changed an excuse to a reason, you have also added a solution.

Your excuse is gone. Now what?

That First Step Could Be Dancin'

It is time to decide on that first step. If you have determined that it is time to get going, begin by deciding what you are going to do. It doesn't have to be too difficult or complicated. Almost everyone likes to dance, so dance. Have fun with it. Dance by yourself in your bedroom, or practice some of those moves you have seen on a music video. It might be fun to pretend you're Elvis, Madonna, or Michael Jackson, all well-known hip-swivelers, or tomorrow's star, or whoever is bustin' the moves on TV at the moment. If you are saying to yourself, "I can't dance," then you are probably right, you can't. The difference is that you can try, and if you aren't very good dancing alone in your bedroom, who cares?

From the Medicine Chest

There are dozens of motivational books, tapes, and videos available. Get a couple, cut out a motivator, and stick in on your bathroom mirror. Get a tape, listen as you walk or drive, and get a video to watch and follow as you begin to exercise.

Health Notes

In his book, *The 7 Habits of Highly Effective People* (Simon & Schuster, 1990), Stephen Covey offers tips to help wipe out negative habits. He says: Be proactive, take the initiative, visualize the end, write how you are going to get there, and make it a priority.

If dancing doesn't do it for you, everyone knows how to walk, so maybe you could start off with making a commitment to walk for 10 minutes every day or every third day. Take along your earphones and some music, and you are close to dancing for 10 minutes. Make a commitment to that 10-minute walk or dance, just like you would another important appointment, and stay with it.

Practice Makes Perfect

You don't think of *not* exercising as a habit, but that's what it is. Based on a very human psychological theory known as the Pleasure Principle, most of us choose unhealthy but enjoyable habits that are hard to abandon for a very human reason: because we enjoy them so much. It might be watching TV or sitting in an easy chair reading, but whatever it is, at the moment it gives you more pleasure than exercising, or at least it seems that way.

Change is a process, so if you are really looking for reasons to not change, you will find them. To move to becoming a person who exercises regularly you need to be convinced that the benefits of making a change exceed the sacrifices.

Psychologists tell us that those who make long-lasting changes in habits go through a well-defined series of stages—*precontemplation, contemplation, preparation, action*, and *maintenance*. These look like a lot of fancy psychological words to describe this process, but here's what they mean:

1. **Precontemplation.** You are thinking that exercise is a good thing. In fact, you know it is a good thing, just not necessarily for you.

2. **Contemplation.** You're thinking about exercising, but you are in that excuse stage. "I'm too busy. I can't afford to join a gym. I'll look into it after my birthday." You will need to weigh the pros and cons so you can decide that the benefits (health) outweigh the cons (feeling lousy).

3. **Preparation.** You've finally decided you are going to walk, take an aerobics class, learn to play golf, or swim. You get a new bathing suit or some shorts and some sunscreen. You've picked a route and are looking forward to admiring the neighbor's flowers along the way, or you've checked out the local aerobics program at the community center or the Y and you have the money to pay for the classes. You are taking the action necessary to begin. You're excited and ready to go. Just getting ready will make you feel more in control. It will strengthen your resolve and give you confidence that you can follow through.

4. **Action.** Whatever you have decided to do, you will need positive thoughts, beliefs, and some behavioral techniques to restructure your mental attitude to make the present "just thinking about it" become reality. (Some action tips follow shortly.)

5. **Maintenance.** Learn from your mistakes and cope with momentary lapses. If you blame yourself because you missed a day or two, it will damage your confidence. But if you keep your perspective and have a positive explanation, you are more likely to return to the good habits you are establishing.

When it comes to following the fourth step, Action, here are some specifics to get you started:

- Make a personal, specific list of what you expect to gain, especially the immediate benefits.

- Set a date to begin, and go public with that date. Once you tell your family and friends that you are going to exercise, and you have waited patiently until they stopped laughing, you have reinforced your commitment. The last thing you want to do is give them a chance to laugh at you again when you don't follow through. You sure don't want to hear, in that gloating tone that is so annoying, "I told you so. I told you you wouldn't keep it up," when you quit.

- Take personal responsibility. The only person in charge of getting you to exercise is you.

- Establish your goals. Outline some doable short-term goals for yourself.

♦ Establish how you will reward yourself. It could be any small item such as a new lipstick, a brightly colored comb, or a groovy T-shirt. Now you have something to work toward.

♦ List a few of the healthier behaviors that will replace the old unhealthy ones.

♦ Change your environment. You can make it easier by avoiding your old habit cues. If you regularly plunk down in front of TV when you get home, don't. Make some small change that will interrupt these cues. If you head for the refrigerator for a little snack or a cold beer as soon as you walk in the house, don't. Decide before you hit the front door what you are going to do that will change your regular triggers.

♦ Get support. Sometimes family and friends can be very supportive, and some of them may like things just the way they are. Recognize the differences and get reinforcement from those people who will sincerely help you to focus on changing. Go places where people talk about how to perform different sports. No, that doesn't mean go to the sports bar where they are just watching people play sports on a big-screen TV. Take a beginner's tennis class or go to the gym and socialize with some of the people there who are just starting out, too.

 Wellness Words

Becoming aware and starting to pay attention is **precontemplation.** It is the moment of truth that makes the problem real. **Contemplation** is beginning to think about change. Beginning to form a game plan, and looking at what is needed to make the change work is **preparation. Action** is beginning to do whatever is necessary to make change. **Maintenance** is finding a new identity and avoid lapses.

Hey Sloopy, Habits Hang On

Habits are strange things, and we all have them—some good, some bad, some neutral. Some studies suggest that in order for the old habit to be extinguished so that you can replace it with a new habit, you must repeat the new one every day for 21 days in a row. Psychologists talk about extinguishing a habit, snuffing it out, and smothering it, and what they actually mean is that you are going to overlay the old bad habit, the one you don't want (couch potatoing) by overlaying it with something more powerful (exercising) until it is simply extinguished. That way, you aren't focusing on the thing you no longer want to do, which actually keeps it as the focal point of your attention. Instead, you are focusing on the new good behavior while the other just melts or fades away.

Why not plan to walk for 10 minutes or 30 minutes or whatever you believe you can do to get started? Don't be unrealistic or dramatic, like deciding you will run a 10K tomorrow morning when you haven't moved too far from the refrigerator for weeks, because that is setting yourself up to become easily demoralized. Then it becomes too easy to say, "I knew it wouldn't work for me." When that happens it is so easy to give up prematurely and slide right back into the old, comfortable habit. Even if you don't stay with it after a couple of days, that isn't failure. That was just your first practice round. Back your goal down a bit and start again.

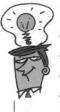

Health Notes

According to the National Institute on Aging, if exercise were a prescription drug, it would be the most widely prescribed medication.

From the Medicine Chest

◆ Keep setting new goals.

◆ Focus on performance.

◆ Use positive self-talk.

◆ Reward positive behavior.

Write It Down to Keep It Up

Next, write it down. No, not just "I will walk 10 minutes every other day" or "I will show up at the gym frequently." Write out the time and the place and any other detail that will make it possible to measure your achievement, and that will make it possible for you to take pleasure in having accomplished it. You might even leave space at the end of each item to write out, "I did it!" so that you can look over your schedule and see yourself accomplishing that positive goal over and over again. When you reward yourself, write it down. We all need an "Atta boy" every once in a while, and even if it isn't a big leap, it's a step, that first step, and a step in the right direction.

Tell Your Friends and Family and Then Step Back!

Before you start your exercise regime, it is a good idea to figure out what situations or people will make making a change more difficult.

Doris, a receptionist in a busy law office, says, "Trying to get rid of an old habit and forming a new one is something like joining a therapy group. It takes the right kind of energy. I'm pretty fond of some of my old habits; they're like old friends. I just don't want to let them go. I'm a little afraid how I will feel about doing something new.

"There are places I go frequently that make me think about eating or drinking or just sitting around laughing with pals instead of working out.

"I have friends and family who laughed when I said I was going to work out—those who knew how often I had made the same old New Year's resolutions and then didn't follow through for very long, and those who don't want to see me change. There are lots of obstacles along the way.

"My friend Lois and I used to meet every morning at a coffee shop right next to where we work for coffee and doughnuts—that's right, doughnuts. We'd spend about 15 minutes griping, gossiping, and eating. When I told her I wanted to start working out in the morning instead of meeting at the coffee shop, and then maybe get some new clothes, she was upset. I realize a couple of things happened. She wasn't motivated to exercise just because I was; she wanted things to stay just the way they were. She was afraid I would try to get her to give up doughnuts, too. We wouldn't have our time to gripe and visit together, and she was afraid she would lose me as friend.

"I have another group of buddies and we all used to go to a local pub for a drink or two after work. I had to decide how valuable that was to me, whether or not I could discipline myself to just stay for half an hour, and what it would mean to those relationships when I began to leave early.

"I know now that even though I love Lois and my other friends, and I still do, when you want to change and the idea is threatening in some way to those around you, you have to be ready for their resistance. There are friends who will support and encourage you, but you have to get ready for the saboteurs, you have to have a strategy already in mind. You have to get prepared, or they will do what they can to disrupt your plan."

Take Your Finger Off the Trigger

We all have triggers, each and every one of us. They are a part of human behavior.

The concept of triggers, unconscious prompts for a behavior or a habit, has been around for almost 150 years. A trigger elicits a known response, so before you start, knowing or recognizing your triggers can go a long way to defusing them or increasing their power, depending on what kind they are and if you want to keep them.

Doris knows that just by going into the doughnut shop, she will smell them and perhaps be tempted to eat one—or several. She also knows that Lois isn't ready to change and will try to prevent her from changing, too.

She knows that by entering the pub she will be tempted to have several drinks and then stay longer than she really should. Then she will be too tired, or she will convince herself that she is too tired, to exercise the next morning.

She also knows that when she gets out her headphones and a tape that she really likes the night before, she has preprogrammed herself to walk when she gets up in the morning. She also knows that she is more likely to walk if things are ready and waiting than if she has to look for her stuff early in the morning.

Doris knows that once Lois realizes that the friendship isn't lost, the two of them can walk and talk with a to-go coffee in their hands. The friendship will last, and maybe she will influence her friend to make some good changes, too.

Doris knows that if she announces when she gets to the pub that she must leave in half an hour because she is taking a class, meeting her mother, or taking care of the neighbor's dog, her friends will be prepared that she won't be staying long.

Doris knows that if she goes in with the resolve that she will only have a soft drink, it will be a lot easier to leave.

Doris knows her negative triggers, and she is taking forethought and action to defuse them. She knows that she could avoid them entirely and, depending on how secure she is in her commitment, that is what she may have to do. She knows how to prepare herself to respond to both negative and positive triggers appropriately.

Doris has taken that first step, and although she isn't even out the door yet, she's ready.

Health Notes

Ivan Pavlov (1849–1936), in his famous study of the learning processes of dogs, stated that after a period of training, with a food reward when a bell rang, a dog would eventually salivate at the sound of a bell, even though it was no longer offered any food when it responded. Psychologists now call this type of response to a signal a trigger. When you want to change any behavior, you need to be aware of your negative triggers so you can avoid or defuse them.

Get a New Identity

We all identify ourselves to others with a variety of adjectives: "I'm George's mother. I'm Mary's husband. I'm a manager at XXX Company. I volunteer with Meals on Wheels. I'm the lead singer with XXX. I'm in the computer department at XXX. I write for the XXX newspaper. I'm a repairman with XXX Company." Our occupation is our identifier to new people we meet. "I'm a hygienist, a law clerk, a fireman, a nurse." New people often don't remember your name, but they remember you as the librarian, the grocery checker, the minister, or the letter carrier.

From the Medicine Chest

Remember "No pain, no gain"? The experts dismiss that as an old-fashioned fitness concept now. Instead, they want you to have "Fun in fitness." When you choose to play, you will enjoy your exercise more, you will be more consistent, and you will reduce your stress level while you improve your fitness and health.

Who Is the Real You?

Your real identifiers are the words you say in your head to identify yourself. You know that you are Mary's husband, or the neighbor, or the computer repair guy, but when you think of yourself and your identity, those identifiers are not the ones you use when you start that mental lecture to yourself about something you did or didn't do. When the boss is angry with you for some minor infraction, the words used to tell you about it take hold. Who hasn't been told by a parent or a teacher or a boss something similar to "How could you be so stupid, careless, thoughtless, reckless, inconsiderate, self-ish, or conceited?" You've heard something similar at some time in your life. Just fill in the blank. Maybe you are one of the millions of people who have been told by a cranky parent, "You'll never amount to anything!" or "Clean up your room, you lazy good-for-nothing." Deep down in your subconscious, your mind embraces that picture of yourself and all of a sudden, you know it is true. Forever.

Lazy, fat, chubby, sloppy, careless, boring. Sometimes you only have to hear or think it once for it to become real.

MLK Identified Millions ... of "Somebodies"

Martin Luther King Jr., in a famous sermon, helped people challenge that kind of self-destructive thinking, the permanent internalizing of a negative identifier. He encouraged people to believe in themselves and say, *"I am somebody."* Millions of small children who had been taught early that they were nobody were able, with those three words, to realize that they were worthwhile and have been encouraged to say daily, "I am somebody." A somebody who deserved to be loved, who deserved to learn, who deserved a chance to realize her dreams. Who knows how many young lives have been changed for the better by those three words.

Maybe the other kids didn't choose you for their team. Maybe you fumbled the ball a couple times. Maybe you were growing fast and stumbled over your own feet. All these things can contribute to a self-identification as someone who doesn't participate well in sports or activities that involve the expenditure of physical energy. You certainly don't want to be stuck with a name given to you by some other dumb kids a decade or more ago.

If any of these identities sound familiar, now is the time to replace them.

If your self-identity includes some of those negative classifications such as *lazy* or *couch potato*, you have some work to do. You will have to start thinking of yourself as what you want to be. Now is the time to begin to tell yourself that you are a power walker, dancer, tennis player, golfer, or mountain climber. Create a new mental image of yourself and then make it happen.

Belief vs. Behavior

If you believe that you can never stick to an exercise regime for any of a dozen reasons, that thought will become a self-fulfilling prophecy, and something will have to change, either your belief or your behavior. Your belief and the way you behave must be in harmony. If they aren't, you will give up one or the other.

However, the exact opposite is also true. If you have finally realized that by just taking that first step on your journey toward wellness that you can become a person who exercises, you are embarking on a wellness trip.

Leon Festinger's *cognitive dissonance* theory states that there is a basic need for each of us to seek consistency among our thoughts (i.e., beliefs, opinions). When there is inconsistency between attitudes and behaviors, it creates an internal conflict. Eventually, it becomes necessary for us to make some kind of a change in either our thinking or our behavior in order to eliminate that internal discord and find peace with the return of mental harmony.

The police know the meaning of the cognitive dissonance theory. They realize they can't put someone out under cover for long periods of time and expect them to pretend to be one of the bad guys without it affecting their thinking and their behavior. A good undercover cop must act real so the crooks will accept the officer as one of their own. By buying into the mindset of the criminal, spending time with them, and doing some of the things they do, it becomes fairly easy to identify with them and begin to adopt their thinking. Police departments have to bring their officers in regularly and give them other assignments to prevent them from accepting that false identity as their real one and eventually becoming a criminal.

Wellness Words

First proposed by Leon Festinger in 1957, the theory of **cognitive dissonance** explains the principle that people's beliefs and behavior must be consistent.

Alcoholics Anonymous is another organization that knows and understands this concept. Many who come to their meetings because they sincerely want to stop abusing alcohol show up intoxicated. A member says, "We know that happens often. It is what happens next that matters. They will either accept the program and stop drinking, or they will continue to drink and stop coming. They simply can't do both."

Behavior vs. Belief

Researchers at Harvard Medical School report that the way older people view themselves is reflected in their walking gaits. Once disease and age-related disability were factored out of the study, it was determined that people who considered themselves wise, astute, and accomplished walk quickly with bounce in their stride. Otherwise healthy people with negative self-images walk more slowly, with less lift and swing to their gait.

Translating the theory of cognitive dissonance into the concept of exercise, you either are a person who works out or you aren't, it is not possible to be both. The responsibility is yours. So take that first step with a swing in your gait and some bounce in your step and start on the road to the new fit you.

The Least You Need to Know

◆ The first step toward becoming a person who exercises regularly is made by turning excuses into legitimate reasons and finding solutions for those reasons.

◆ The Pleasure Principle keeps you locked into the same old bad habits—ones you enjoy.

◆ The five steps to turn bad habits into good ones are precontemplation, contemplation, preparation, action, and maintenance. They will assist you in turning those bad habits into good ones as painlessly as possible.

◆ Looking for supportive people in your life and planning ahead to deal with friends and family who don't want you to change can make a big difference in whether or not you reach and keep your exercise goal.

◆ Cognitive dissonance theory states there is a tendency to make your behavior and attitudes consistent, and you need to apply this theory to exercise to make it work for you.

Run, Walk, or Ride—Just Choose Your Weapon

In This Chapter

◆ How to exercise sensibly

◆ Choosing the right workout for you

◆ The right equipment

Aerobic exercise and anaerobic exercise are the two basic forms of exercise. Each produces different effects on the body, and the body needs them both. Here is a brief definition of these two types of exercise:

◆ **Aerobic exercise** involves continuous activity so that your lungs work harder to bring in oxygen and your heart works harder to pump blood to your muscles. The word *aerobic* literally means "with oxygen." This type of exercise can be maintained continuously for a long period of time. It trains the heart, lungs, and cardiovascular system to process and deliver oxygen to the body. Aerobic exercise promotes cardiovascular fitness by raising your pulse to a slowly increasing targeted level. Walking, swimming, and dancing are examples of aerobic exercises. It is recommended that you exercise within your target heart rate range three times a week.

◆ **Anaerobic exercise** causes a metabolic process to take place in your muscles where it burns fat and energy 70 percent more quickly than in aerobic exercise. The word *anaerobic* literally means "without oxygen." Anaerobic exercise builds muscle strength and endurance. Weight training, baseball, and flexibility training such as yoga are examples of anaerobic exercises. Anaerobic oxidation implies that the process is so vigorous that there is not enough oxygen present to complete the metabolic process in the muscles. Resistance against a weight, such as in weight lifting, is a prime example of anaerobic work. Even though a number of activities such as football, baseball, or tennis may be played for several hours, most of it is aerobic and the anerobic activity generally takes place in short, perhaps three-minute intervals during the game. In baseball, for example, that would be the time when the batter swings the bat and then makes a brief all-out sprint to first base. A cyclist would experience short bursts of anaerobic exercise during the effort it takes to pedal the bike up a steep hill. Even golf, if the player carries his own clubs and drives the ball a long distance, can be considered to include some anaerobic exercise. Weight lifting is the most well known of all the anaerobic exercises.

In this chapter, we'll discuss these forms of exercise and how to prepare your mind and body to incorporate them into your daily life. Let's start out talking about aerobic exercise, which you measure by calculating your heart rate as you exercise.

Your Heart and Exercise

Any beginning exerciser needs to know how to avoid stressing his or her heart by trying to do too much too rapidly. When you work out, it is important to work at an intensity level that is correct for you. Your target heart rate isn't one single number, but a range of rates or beats per minute that are safe for you to reach during exercise. Depending on your level of fitness, knowing what your pulse rate range should be so that you can exercise safely and still receive the maximum cardiovascular benefits is the reason for calculating your target heart rate range. For most healthy people, the American Heart Association recommends an exercise target heart rate ranging from 50 to 75 percent of your maximum heart rate.

Whatever aerobic exercise you choose to do, it should be strenuous enough to make your heart beat somewhere within the range of its target rate during your workout.

CAUTION 911!

Each year, thousands of people injure themselves by pushing too hard, advancing too early, and not paying attention to their body when it says enough. This is about winning the wellness game, not a sporting competition. You don't need to win the race or the contest, lift the heaviest weights, or ride your bike the farthest. Listen to your body, and you won't become an exercise dropout because you injured yourself and had to quit. If you have a pre-existing injury or medical condition, consider that before you undertake any new exercise regime.

If you're interested in being completely accurate, you could buy a heart rate monitor, but it isn't necessary. Instead, use this tried-and-true method of calculating your heart rate.

First find your carotid artery. You will find it by putting your index finger on the side of your neck between the middle of your collarbone and your jaw. Then either count the beats for 1 minute to be most accurate, or count for 10 seconds and multiply by 6.

Hearts can only beat about 220 per minute for men and 226 for women.

Your target heart rate range is the one at which you can exercise *safely* and get the most cardiovascular benefits. As your fitness level increases, you can increase your target heart rate range.

To calculate a sustained target heart rate for yourself, subtract your age from the 220 for men or the 226 for women, and then calculate a percentage of that amount.

Example: 220

A 35-year-old man: −35 = 185 × 50 percent = 92

The lower end of his target heart rate is 92 beats per minute.

185 × 60 percent = 111

The upper end of his target heart rate is 111 beats per minute.

His target range is anywhere between 92 and 111 beats per minute. Someone who is just starting to work out should keep his heart rate in the lower range. Once he is comfortable there, he can increase the intensity of his workout.

Example: 226

A 50-year-old woman: −50 = 176 × 50 percent = 88

The lower end of her target heart rate is 88 beats per minute.

176 × 60 percent = 106

The upper end of her target heart rate is 106 beats per minute. A woman who is just starting to exercise should keep her heart rate in the lower range until she is comfortable there. Then she can increase the intensity of her workout.

Targeting Your Heart Rate

Take a look at the following categories of exercise and their target heart rates. During a typical exercise session, you should measure your heart rate several times. It's especially important to warm up all of your muscles—including your heart—and then to cool down before you stop altogether. Aim for the listed target heart rate ranges during each stage of exercise every time you work out.

Warm-up, cool down, and beginner rates: 50 to 60 percent of maximum heart rate

This heart rate is good for warming up and for those just starting a fitness program. Keeping your heart rate in this zone for 15 to 30 minutes will assist you in decreasing body fat and lowering both blood pressure and cholesterol levels. It has a very low risk of injury, and 85 percent of the calories burned in this zone are from fats.

Working out: 60 to 70 percent of maximum heart rate

This heart rate is good for any workout. It will assist you in decreasing body fat and lowering both blood pressure and cholesterol levels. Eighty-five percent of the calories burned in this zone are from fats.

Endurance: 70 to 80 percent of maximum heart rate

Working out at this heart rate will improve your cardiovascular and respiratory abilities and will increase the size and strength of your heart. If you are training for a distance run or any of the other sustained exercise activities, this is an excellent maximum rate. This workout burns more calories, with 50 percent of them being from fats.

Pro: 80 to 90 percent of maximum heart rate

Working at this heart rate is good for serious athletes such as cross-country skiers and mountain climbers. This rate will improve your ability to use oxygen and improve your cardio respiratory abilities. Endurance and the ability to fight fatigue will improve. It will burn more calories, but only 15 percent of them will be fats.

You probably noticed that when you reach the upper limits of heart rates, you burn less fat. The reason for this is that you begin to burn glucose or sugar, which is immediately available, rather than the fats you have stored.

Everybody Stretch!

No matter what exercise you choose, you should stretch out before your routine. Even those golfers, who ride in carts and walk only a few feet to lightly tap a ball into the cup, need to warm up and stretch in order to avoid injury. Your body has a natural lubricant, called synovial fluid, in all your joints, and it needs a chance to spread across your joints to oil them up for action. It works just like the warm oil in your car, preventing parts from grinding against each other.

Stretching also helps you achieve your maximum range of motion and prevents lactic acid, a byproduct of carbohydrate metabolism, necessary to provide energy to fuel your muscles, from building-up in the muscles. Lactic acid is known to cause fatigue, muscle soreness, and painful muscle cramps.

Cold, tight muscles don't work smoothly, either. A sudden start or jerky motion of a tight muscle is just asking for a tear or damage to the tendons or cartilage.

A good warm-up should be specific to your sport. If you are lifting weights, start out by lifting some lighter weights. If you are walking, start out at a slower pace, and once you are feeling warm, gently stretch your muscles before you really get moving. You will perform better and avoid injuries.

From the Medicine Chest

Strolling is sightseeing, not walking. It is *not* an aerobic workout. Putting your heart into something higher than its resting rate is *absolutely necessary* for you to get *any* aerobic benefits from walking.

Before You Choose Your Weapons

You can, of course, choose activities that require very expensive equipment and go out and outfit yourself with all that you need. You could even buy a polo pony, but before you get yourself too excited about some exotic sport, you probably need to learn a little something about it and then do something to get in shape for that exciting experience in your future.

You can probably run, glide, ride, or slide in the stuff you already own, like some shorts, sweatpants, a comfortable T-shirt or two, and a hat. The one thing you need, if you don't already own them, is a pair of well-fitting and supporting shoes. Until then, hold off on putting a down payment on that fancy sailboat.

From the Medicine Chest

If you are 10 pounds overweight, climbing stairs puts four times the normal amount of stress a person of normal weight puts on the ligaments and tendons of his knees. It is like picking up a 40-pound box and carrying it with you every time you climb. More than four million people seek medical treatment for knee ailments annually. If you are having knee problems, consider losing weight by simply walking before you consider using equipment such as stair-climbers or performing any climbing-type exercise.

Now Choose Your Weapons

There is an endless list of exercises that you can choose to do. The most important criterion is their fun quotient: The more fun you find them, the more likely you are to continue to do them. Another way to prevent your exercise from becoming drudgery is to alter your choices.

For example, you could walk one day, ride your bike another, swim a third, and if you already have some equipment or some skills, play tennis, look for a pickup game of basketball, or roller blade.

And you don't have to get fancy: There are lots of aerobic exercises you already know how to do. Walking, gardening, swimming, jogging, dancing, skating, rowing, ice or roller skating, and skiing are some activities you might be familiar with. Any of them provides excellent aerobic conditioning.

Or maybe you could explore an activity you know very little about but might like to learn. The list is probably endless, but here are a few you might want to consider: artificial wall climbing, surfing, softball, snowshoeing, cardio kickboxing, touch football, and fencing.

Fortunately, there are also endless supplies of motivating and instructional videocassettes you can rent for a couple of dollars. There are dozens of books with illustrations on how to proceed when you want to try something new. A look at the magazine section of your local bookstore may surprise you. You can probably count at least 35 fitness magazines, each one devoted to a single topic such as running or weight lifting. If you think you are self-motivated enough to begin on your own, you might want to give some of them a try by renting a video or reading a magazine before you venture into a class.

Another way to keep your exercise fun is to do it with someone. You may have a friend willing to walk every morning. Maybe you know someone you could play tennis with, and there is always the possibility that if you join a gym or take a class, you may make a new friend, someone already interested in staying healthy and participating with you in healthful activities. You might even fall in love—you just never know.

CAUTION **911!** _____

Don't fall for a fad. Fads come and go; that is why they are known as fads. Some fads are good; some are ridiculous. But learning about some may expose you to new ideas and new experiences, and if you want to try some of them that may be a good thing. If you read an article or see some expert on TV that piques your interest, you might want to give one a try, providing you get in good condition first, particularly some of the more strenuous exercise. Just like anything else, do it in moderation until you know whether or not it is right and good for you.

Try Walking!

Walking—yes just plain walking—is one of the safest and most effective form of aerobic exercise. If you walk for 30 minutes at a moderate pace (about 50 to 60 percent of your target heart rate) three or four times a week, you'll be giving your heart, your body, and your mind a terrific workout. Researchers at California State University say that just 10 minutes of brisk walking or power walking will elevate your mood and energy and for 1 to 2 hours afterward.

In addition to regular walking, there are two other types of exercise in the walking category: race walking and power walking. Race walking is that funny-looking way of walking you see every once in a while on TV. The exaggerated arm movements and overstriding of race-walking has been linked to many injuries. It is difficult to learn and actually hard on your lower back.

Power walking is walking at a brisk pace. Walk 1 mile in 12 to 15 minutes, and you are a power walker. All you have to do when you walk is pick up the pace and increase your distance and frequency, and you are a power walker. Saying "I power walk" sounds a lot more impressive than just telling folks you've been out taking a walk, doesn't it?

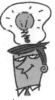

From the Medicine Chest

Walking burns more calories than running. Five miles at a brisk pace burns 530 calories, compared to 480 calories for jogging. The reason: Walkers take more steps and use their arms more.

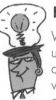

From the Medicine Chest

When you power walk, use good posture and don't add hand or ankle weights because they will alter your stride. Look straight ahead, not at the ground. Bend your arms slightly and don't swing your elbows higher than your breastbone. Resist the urge to increase your stride. Instead, if you want to go faster, take smaller, faster steps.

Exercise Alternatives

There are some exercise routines that are more enjoyable than others. It makes sense to find something that you like to do if you plan to stick with exercising regularly. If you find that tennis or running or trampolining just isn't for you, you might want to try some of the alternatives. A number of people simply fall in love with unusual things such as yoga or tai chi, but they wouldn't know about them without giving them a trial run. So try it, you might like it.

- ◆ **Yoga.** In his book *Introduction to Yoga Principles* (University Books, 1966), Sachindra Kumar Majumdar tells us that yoga originated in India more than 4,000 years ago. The most common method taught in the West today is known as Hatha Yoga, which concentrates on both physical health and mental well-being. It consists mainly of stretching and bending poses performed very slowly in time with your breathing. During a session the exercises are done in sitting, standing, and lying positions, all followed at the end in a period of relaxation. Those who practice yoga become stronger and more flexible, and they say that the breathing and period of relaxation provides them with a stress-reducing feeling of serenity.

◆ **Tai chi.** Although it looks very easy, tai chi, an exercise form developed in China, is actually quite challenging. A version of the martial art of kung fu, tai chi is a series of slow flowing movements with the feet in positions that ensure perfect balance. These movements are coordinated with the breathing of the participant, and the control of the breath in rhythm with the movements aims at improving general well-being.

◆ **Qigong.** In *The Way of Qigong* (Ballantine Books, 1997), Kenneth Cohen reports that qigong and tai chi both originated in China. Qigong's vigorous movement takes the body through a series of postures as though performing a dance. The aim of qigong is for the individual to be active on the outside and through controlled breathing and become quiet on the inside. It uses movements that have names that elicit mental pictures of the movements such as Swimming Dragon and Standing Crane.

Unlike yoga, both tai chi and qigong are performed standing only, perfecting balance. Both disciplines are aimed at achieving health by opening the pathways within the body through which each person's energy flows.

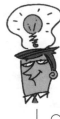

From the Medicine Chest

You can buy all the equipment you see in your local gym for use at home: rowing machines, elliptical motion trainers, stair-climbers, gravity boots, rebounders, indoor skiing machines, free weights, pulse meters, and computerized blood pressure read-outs. You can even own a stationary bike called a Lifecycle that will flash information about how you are doing while you use it, like your maximum oxygen uptake. Owning your own can cost you several thousand dollars.

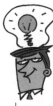

From the Medicine Chest

Muscle size and development varies between men and women and is dependent on the hormone testosterone. While women do produce a very small amount of this hormone, men have 10 times as much. Because of their low level of testosterone, there is no need for women to worry about "bulking up" from weight lifting.

◆ **Pilates.** Allan Menezes outlines the method of Joseph Pilates in his book *Joseph H. Pilates' Techniques of Physical Conditioning* (Hunter House, 2000). Pilates devised a method of returning people to health through a system he called contrology. It is a system of nonweight-bearing, no-impact exercise based on strengthening the "core" muscles of the abdomen. It lengthens, defines, and sculpts muscles and has long been the preferred exercise of dancers. Although many physical therapists use elaborate Pilates equipment that assists in elongating the muscles, there are also Pilates mat classes where the weight of your own body is used to correcting imbalances.

◆ **Spinning.** www.spinning.com explains that in the 1980s world-class cyclist Jonathan Goldberg, a.k.a. "Johnny G.," created a unique indoor stationary cycling program. Participants wear heart monitors while they go through a series of five movements around a series of training sessions that include endurance, strength, interval, racing, and recovery. Spinners use specially designed stationary bikes, and many gyms now include spinning as part of regularly offered programs.

◆ **Birkham yoga.** This yoga practice became very popular in Beverly Hills and is presided over by its creator Choudhury Bikram, who bills himself as "Yogi to the Stars." Centers have opened at a variety of spas and locations; you can even find one in Nebraska. Participants perform 90 minutes of athletically demanding yoga postures in a 105-degree heated, specially constructed room. Adherents claim that it increases energy, creates such extreme sweating that will rid your of all your toxins, and at the same time dramatically reduces stress levels.

From the Medicine Chest

American Sports Data, Inc., reports that snow boarding, skateboarding, and wakeboarding—three of the so-called "extreme" sports—were the fasting-growing sports in the last year. During 2000, the number of people participating in snowboarding increased by 51 percent.

Togetherness Fitness

Nancy and Earl are a very busy couple. She has her own catering business, and he is a corporate attorney. She is often out in the evening overseeing the serving of a fancy dinner for several hundred people, and he is frequently away in the office until late at night.

Nancy said, "We began to realize that we weren't spending much time together. When we did have any free time, just so we could get some exercise, I went to an aerobics class and Earl played handball with his buddies at a local sports center.

"We often talked about doing things together, but Earl is taller than I am and outweighs me by almost 100 pounds." Nancy laughed, "I didn't think I was going to win at almost anything we could do together. For a while we rode our bikes on Saturday mornings, but the traffic was terrible, and while we were together, it wasn't possible to talk unless we got the bikes side-by-side."

A neighbor suggested power walking, and they began getting up just half an hour earlier in the morning to walk together.

"At first we were exhausted. We couldn't believe how tough it was. Now we log 30 to 40 miles a week and have walked marathons! The great part is that while we walk early in the morning, we are spending time together and talking every day. It's wonderful."

Earl agreed, "It is so much better to talk things over early in the morning rather than late at night when we are both tired and stressed out with our days' problems. We are closer emotionally and feel more romantic when we see each other in the evening. It certainly has improved our outlook on life and our marriage. It's helping both of us to maintain our weight, and neither one of us has had a cold in months. We have added a little weight lifting, just another 15 minutes, to balance our upper body strength with the lower body strength power walking gives us. I think we both look, well, powerful."

Full Fitness

Aerobic exercise keeps your heart and lungs healthy. Anaerobic exercise builds muscle strength and endurance. Warming up and stretching improve range of motion and flexibility. Doesn't a healthy heart, strong muscles, and flexible body sound like something you would like to have?

Health Notes

The YMCA website reports that there are thousands of Y locations throughout the world, and most have exercise programs. There are local gyms or health clubs with community-sponsored events where you can learn a skill such as tennis or volleyball quite inexpensively. A look in the Yellow Pages in your locale should provide some contact numbers.

The Least You Need to Know

♦ Calculate your target heart rate range, a percentage of the maximum rate of 220 for men and 226 for women minus your age, in order to exercise safely and get the most cardiovascular benefits. Most exercise, such as running, walking, and tennis, is aerobic exercise. It improves your heart, lungs, and cardiovascular system. Anaerobic exercise, in short bursts (about three minutes each) of pushing or pulling against resistance, such as swinging a bat or lifting weights, builds muscle and increases endurance and flexibility.

♦ Some exercise choices and their target heart ranges are better for beginners, endurance, or pro athletes. Walking, tai chi, Pilates, and spinning are some alternative choices you might like to try. Every one can walk, and power walking will get you in great shape.

♦ No matter what exercise you choose and enjoy, everyone needs both cardiovascular and strength training, as well as a warm up and stretches to avoid injury.

Part 4

The Third Pillar—
Stress Management

Now that you've tackled your nutritional and exercise goals, it's time to get a handle on the stresses of your everyday life and learn how to turn them to your advantage. What bugs you may inspire someone else, so it's all about figuring out just what people, circumstances, and events send you over the edge. Once you know that, you can make a sensible game plan for combating stress and making it your ally, not your enemy.

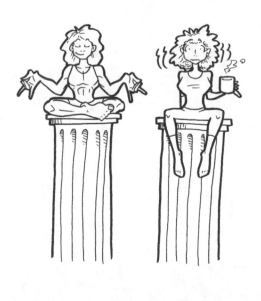

Does Stress Really Cause Illness?

In This Chapter

- ◆ The link between stress and getting sick
- ◆ The top causes of stress
- ◆ The physical signs of stress
- ◆ Fighting fire with fire

When it was first suggested that stress could perhaps be a root cause of disease and illness, the researchers who presented the hypothesis were practically laughed out of the scientific world. Today, thanks to many carefully controlled studies, we know there is a definite link between stress and the development of certain diseases.

Will you automatically get sick just because you're stressed out all the time? No. A lot depends on how you handle stress. If you manage it well, it will not affect your health in the long run. If you let it eat you up, sooner or later the constant assaults of stress-related hormones on your body and immune system will definitely increase your odds of developing an illness or having an accident. In this chapter, we'll explore the connection in some depth.

Does Stress Cause Illness?

Although researchers have firmly established the link between too much stress and an increased risk of illness and accidents, no study has yet proven a direct causal link between stress and any specific illness. So if someone says to you, "Stress causes cancer," that's not exactly right. Stress weakens your immune system and may make it easier for cancer or another disorder to take hold in your body, but it doesn't actually cause disease in the same way that a bacteria or virus or cancer cell does.

Still, long-term stress can lead to a variety of illnesses. The American Institute of Stress says that 43 percent of all American adults suffer some form of adverse health effect due to stress. They also estimate that anywhere from 75 to 90 percent of visits to primary care physicians are for stress-related complaints.

Health Notes

As far back as 55 B.C.E., the ancient Greeks already understood that worry and stress were more a function of your outlook than anything else. The Greek Stoic philosopher, Epictetus, said it well: "Men are disturbed, not by things, but by the principles and notions which they form concerning things." Epictetus said when you can't change something, you can at least change how it makes you feel. That's still good advice today.

Illnesses Linked to Stress

No one knows why one person develops a particular stress-related illness while another person gets another and still a third person stays healthy. Here are a few examples of stress-related illnesses:

- **Cardiovascular disease.** One of the first physical ailments linked directly to stress. Way back in the 1950s, researchers proved that aggressive, hostile, impatient, competitive, temperamental Type-A personalities were much more likely to suffer heart attacks than the laid-back Type-B personalities who took life's little mishaps in stride. Researchers now believe that stress plays a role not only in heart attacks, but also in other forms of cardiovascular disease, including angina, high blood pressure, and cerebrovascular strokes.

- **Gastrointestinal disease.** We've all heard of people with "nervous stomachs" who get a stomachache or throw up when faced with stress. Crohn's disease, irritable bowel syndrome, ulcers, and chronic diarrhea are other manifestations of stress on the digestive system.

◆ **Obesity.** Stress can play a major role in the development of obesity when people treat their stress by overindulging in comforting foods like ice cream and chocolate. Obesity itself is a major risk factor for heart disease, diabetes, and high blood pressure.

◆ **Psychological disorders.** Stress plays a role in depression, panic, and anxiety disorders. Stress can also lead to a dependence on drugs or alcohol as people seek to relieve its symptoms.

◆ **Colds and flu.** Because stress weakens the immune system, people who suffer from chronic stress are much more likely to develop colds, flu, upper respiratory infections, and other opportunistic infections upon exposure.

◆ **Cancer.** No definitive link between cancer and stress has ever been established clinically, but many cancer sufferers believe in such a link and trace the onset of their cancer to a particularly difficult time in their lives. The concept of a "Type-C" or "cancer personality," which portrays cancer patients as typically weak, ineffectual people who are habitually victimized by others, has mercifully been put to rest.

Why Does Stress Make Me Feel So Bad?

Your body perceives stress as a physical emergency. When you are feeling stressed, your cerebral cortex sends a signal to the center of your brain, your hypothalamus, which, in turn signals your nervous system to make changes in response to the stress. Your heart rate, respiration, and blood pressure increase rapidly. Your hands sweat, your pupils dilate, and your hearing acuity increases. Blood and oxygen are diverted away from your extremities to the large muscles that could help you run away from a physical threat or stand and fight it. All these changes occur as a result of chemical signals sent by your adrenal glands, which pump adrenaline, epinephrine, norepinephrine, and cortisol through your bloodstream. These chemicals inhibit digestion as well as the immune and inflammatory responses. In other words, stress disrupts your vital bodily functions in order to prepare you to meet a potentially deadly external threat. At least, that's what it was originally designed to do.

CAUTION

911!

Are you too stressed? Place your fingertips against the side of your neck. If your fingers feel as warm as your neck, you're fine. If they feel cold, you're stressed. When your body feels stressed, it diverts warming oxygenated blood to its central core, thereby lowering the temperature in your fingertips. The colder your fingertips, the more stressed out you are. If your fingers are cold, start one of your stress management techniques right away to get the blood flowing again.

This reaction may be well and good when you actually have to run or fight. But when stress is unrelenting and your body never gets a chance to use the stress chemicals you keep producing, you reach a state where you are awash in these powerful chemicals on a more or less constant basis, and that can make you feel pretty bad.

Fight or Flight Is Out of Date

When we were cavemen, the stress reaction served us well. If someone tried to smack you with his club, you went into your fight-or-flight mode as your brain pumped huge amounts of adrenaline into your bloodstream, which meant that you could instantly call upon your body for an extra burst of energy to get away from the danger. During your escape, your body burned off the chemicals it used to trigger your escape. When the danger passed, you settled down to your nice meal of roasted wooly mastodon, and everything went back to normal. Generally speaking, the fight-or-flight reflex was only activated a few times a week, and you used up all the powerful hormones and chemicals the stress response triggered as you responded to the danger.

Contrast that single instance of immediate stress to the chronic stress common today, when a nasty boss, angry spouse, or stubborn child may trigger your stress response dozens of time over the course of a day. Add to that traffic, noise, pollution, money worries, and deadlines, just to name a few, and you can see how modern life has become one long stream of unremitting stress. We get buffeted with stress all day long. It's how we choose to respond to it that can make the difference in how it makes us feel.

Stress Is Costly to Business

The National Safety Council (NSC) estimates that on any given workday, an average of one million employees are absent in the United States due to stress or stress-related problems. Stress may be either job-related, like a bad boss or a bullying co-worker, or brought from home, like financial problems or a child doing poorly in school. But no matter where the stress originates, it is costly. It not only causes increased absenteeism, but also negatively affects productivity, interoffice relationships and team-building, and leads to increased employee turnover and a greater risk of on-the-job accidents.

According to the NSC, stress costs American employers an average of $80 billion a year. That's an awfully steep price, but it is still not as high as the cost to the individuals who are trying to cope with stress. The price they pay in terms of their health and happiness

> **Health Notes**
>
> Just in case you don't buy the idea that stress costs businesses big bucks, look at the *Exxon Valdez* and Three Mile Island incidents. In both cases, the people responsible for the accidents were under multiple stressors, including sleep deprivation, overwork, inadequate training, and other job-related stresses. The direct cost of cleanup for these two incidents was a little more than $3 billion.

is almost incalculable, which is one more good reason to learn how to manage your stress now.

Stress and Burnout

When people suffer from unrelieved stress over a long period of time, they may develop a condition known as *burnout*. One of the most prevalent characteristics of burnout is a loss of motivation. Sufferers may show apathy and a complete lack of interest in the events and people around them. The productivity of burned-out employees may plummet as they become progressively detached from their jobs, their co-workers, and their surroundings. They may begin to question their own worth to the company or the value of the job they are doing.

Burnout has become such a significant problem for American businesses that an entire industry has sprung up to help employers cope with the problem. If you suspect that you are suffering from job burnout, ask your supervisor if your company provides any treatment or interventions to help you recover your enthusiasm.

Wellness Words

Burnout is the exhaustion of physical and emotional strength accompanied by a near-total lack of motivation that usually results from prolonged stress or frustration.

Stress Causes Accidents

Stress plays a big role in workplace accidents. According to the National Safety Council, anywhere from 60 to 80 percent of on-the-job mishaps are stress-related. Stress is particularly dangerous for people in hazardous professions like the building trades and manufacturing because it causes inattentiveness. One careless move on a fast-moving production line can cause a serious or even life-threatening accident, which is why companies spend hundreds of thousands of dollars annually researching stress in the workplace and looking for solutions.

The best solution lies within you. You are the best judge of how much you can handle, and you're the only one who knows with any certainty when you are approaching your breaking point. There are many ways for you to recognize your stress and defuse it before it becomes something more serious.

The Many Causes of Stress

We discussed in Chapter 3, "The Four Pillars of Wellness," how there are actually two kinds of stress: good stress, or eustress, and bad stress, or distress. Both can have detrimental effects on the body if they are not managed properly.

What causes stress? There are three basic causes:

- ◆ **Environmental stress** can be caused by the weather, noise, traffic, pollution, stressful interpersonal relationships at work or home, a demanding schedule, inadequate shelter, deadlines, and overwork.

- ◆ **Physical stress** can be caused by a poor diet, lack of exercise, weight problems, sleep deprivation, health problems, chronic illness, hormonal changes such as those brought about by pregnancy or menopause, growing older, and accidents.

- ◆ **Psychological stress** can be caused by anxiety, worry, fear, insecurity, self-esteem issues, being a victim of a bully or harasser, or any other emotions that make a person feel overwhelmed, helpless, and unable to cope.

Take Control

We may not have much control over what happens in our environment or inside our bodies, but we do have some control. For example, if your boss has a foul temper and uses you for a scapegoat, you can quit and find another job or ask for a transfer to another department. If you can't stand cold weather but are stuck in a snowy climate, it will help you deal with that stress if you start working on a plan to move to a warmer climate when you are able. The point is, no matter how bad your situation, you are not entirely powerless. With a little thought, you should be able to come up with some creative solutions for stress relief.

If you suffer from arthritis or some other chronic condition, you can investigate exercise and pain management programs that will give you better control over the condition.

As for psychological stress, that's where we have the most control. We can control our own thoughts and reactions. All it takes is a determination to do it. Controlling and channeling our reactions to both external and internal stimuli is at the heart of effective stress management.

And remember, if you tell yourself that you *cannot* make a change when really you can, you are creating additional stress by your refusal to look at possible solutions to your problems.

Depending on how you respond, receiving a big raise and promotion could be just as stressful to you and just as damaging to your body as getting fired from your job. It's all a matter of how you look at things.

From the Medicine Chest

Stress results not from what is happening to you, but from your perception of what is happening to you. If you always feel negative, like the world is against you or that bad things are always happening to you, then you will feel a lot of stress. On the other hand, if you have a positive outlook and have learned to incorporate exercise, breathing, journaling, and other effective stress management tools into your life, you can probably handle a lot of stress without experiencing undue physical or psychological effects.

Watch Out for the Small Things

We all know that big life events like the death of a spouse or close family member, the breakdown of a marriage or important romantic relationship, the loss of a job, a serious injury or illness, and even retirement can be big stressors. But the little stressors can add up to big problems, too.

Let's imagine you forgot to pick up your spouse's dry cleaning and now he's angry because the dry cleaner is closed and he doesn't have a clean shirt for the next day. You start to cook dinner, feeling inadequate and guilty as your husband starts to yell at you again. You rush back into the den to take up the fight while your unattended skillet full of hot oil catches fire. You rush back to the kitchen but because you're so upset, you don't think to use the fire extinguisher right next to the stove. Instead, you throw a glass of water on the fire, which causes it to spread explosively, burning your hands and arms in the process.

Sound unlikely? It happens every single day, because we all try to juggle too many things, way more than what the human mind and body was designed to accommodate at once.

A better way would have been to sincerely apologize to your spouse, offer to launder and press a shirt at home that evening, and refuse to engage in any ongoing discussions about the situation. You can keep little stressors from developing into major problems simply by putting a lid on it. If someone is baiting you to argue, simply walk away and take 10 deep breaths, or perform some of the other stress management techniques we discuss in Chapter 18, "What Are Your Stress Triggers?" Just don't play the game—you'll be healthier and happier for it.

Are You Your Own Worst Enemy?

Sometimes the stress we feel comes from inside our own heads. We can have the most wonderful spouse in the world, ideal children, a dream job, and yet we persist in feeling like the victim. If this is the case, the stress you feel is probably *self-generated*.

Some of the contributing causes to self-generated stress may include the following:

Wellness Words

Self-generated stress is any stress that results from an internal rather than an external pressure and is generally based on faulty perceptions and thinking.

- Perfectionism
- A desire to please
- A self-imposed pressure to excel
- Excessive self-criticism
- An inability to accept sincere compliments
- An unreasonable desire for perfect control in every situation
- Obsession with personal appearance
- The belief that a lack of control is a sign of weakness and failure

If you recognize any of these characteristics in yourself, most or all of your stress may be self-generated. Self-generated stress can be one of the most difficult kinds of stress to overcome. It's almost as if you are caught inside a loop of negative thinking inside your own head. To make sure you are not dealing with another problem like anxiety disorder, seek professional help if you are struggling with a lot of self-generated stress.

What Stress Does to Your Body

Stress affects your body in many ways. The physical signs are most apparent. Let's review the symptoms we listed in Chapter 3.

Physical signs:

- Difficulty falling asleep or staying asleep
- Digestive upsets, nausea, bloating, cramping, and diarrhea
- Racing heart
- Tension or migraine headaches
- A feeling of tightness in the chest
- Generalized body aches or backache
- Unusual fatigue
- Change in eating habits

Stress can also make you perspire or tremble, give you a feeling of butterflies in your stomach, make your mouth and throat feel dry, and even make you urinate more frequently. Now let's review the emotional symptoms of stress from Chapter 3.

Emotional or psychological signs:

- A racing mind and the inability to settle down and concentrate
- Forgetfulness
- Paranoid or illogical thinking
- Irritable and easily distracted
- Impatient
- Unusually depressed or anxious
- Easily angered
- Feelings of isolation and loneliness
- Increase in use of alcohol and tobacco products
- Inappropriate use of prescription or over-the-counter drugs
- Use of illicit drugs

In addition, you may feel anxious or scared and struggle with feelings of failure and low self-esteem. You may have trouble concentrating because you are so distracted by your worries.

Stress can also produce distinct behavioral changes including over- or undereating, stuttering, bruxism or grinding of the teeth, spontaneous crying for no discernible reason, nervous laughter, and impulsive behavior. It can also increase your risk of having an accident.

If you observe several of these signs in yourself or a close family member, your stress level is getting out of control and your body is reacting in an attempt to manage on its own. Don't let stress rule your life. By taking charge of your stress and choosing a new outlook, you can make your life happier and more fulfilling.

Self-Medication Is *Not* a Good Idea

Some people deal with stress by drinking or taking drugs. The chemicals in alcohol and recreational drugs serve to mask or lessen the symptoms of stress. Dealing with stress by self-medicating in this way is not a good idea. You cannot deal with stress successfully by glossing over its root causes.

Even worse is that these behaviors tend to get worse with time. It takes more and more booze or cocaine to bury the negative feelings associated with stress as time goes on. Indulging in such behaviors only puts you in a downward spiral with nowhere to go.

Other people deal with stress by bingeing on sweets, or gambling, or shopping too much. All of these behaviors are forms of self-medication that allow you to ignore your real underlying problems.

If you are dealing with addictive behavior, chances are that stress relief may be at least one component of the causes for that behavior. If so, you need to get a handle on your self-medication as quickly as possible. Drug and alcohol abuse lead to addiction, bingeing leads to obesity, shopping and gambling lead to indebtedness, and all lead to additional health problems down the road. The time to stop these self-destructive behaviors is now. Get professional help and learn how to manage your stress-related problems in a better, healthier way.

The Least You Need to Know

- ◆ Researchers have established a definite link between ongoing stress and the development of illness.
- ◆ Any major life change, whether good or bad, can cause stress.
- ◆ Stress can produce a variety of physical complaints ranging from headaches to back pain to digestive upsets.
- ◆ Treating your stress with alcohol or drugs just leads to additional problems.

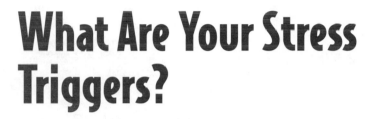

Chapter 18

What Are Your Stress Triggers?

In This Chapter

- ◆ What gets your goat?
- ◆ Figuring out what you can change
- ◆ Fight or flight
- ◆ Hitting the "off" switch

We all react to different stressors; what makes you mad may not so much as ruffle the feathers of your spouse or best friend. Because we humans are an egocentric bunch and tend to believe that everyone else should feel and act exactly as we do, these different reactions to stressful situations can in and of themselves be an additional cause of stress and conflict. In this chapter, we will help you identify your primary stress triggers so that you'll know exactly what sets you off.

Why is this important? Because if you can't identify your own hot buttons, you won't be able to use the information in Chapter 19, "Tools and Techniques to Manage Stress," to manage your stress effectively. If you and your significant other take the "Hot Button" test together (you'll see that soon), you can learn a lot about what sets each of you off and should be able to devise some intelligent alternatives to avoid pressing each other's hot buttons all the time.

Them's Fighting Words

Each of us can remember at least one or two instances in our lives when someone we cared about got unreasonably angry, or at least it seemed unreasonable from our point of view. The recall of such incidents is usually accompanied by numerous jests at the expense of the person who got angry and everyone has a good time except the poor person who's the butt of the joke.

The point is, whatever got the person angry in the first place doesn't matter, because at the time of the incident their reaction was authentic and true to their personality and circumstances.

Now think about what gets you worked up. Is it traffic? Your spouse's overspending? Your employee's habitual tardiness? Your losing battle with your expanding waistline? What makes you feel sad? A death in the family? Losing your job? Financial problems?

> **Health Notes**
>
> Way back in 1967, Drs. Thomas H. Holmes and Richard H. Rahe devised a now-famous test to predict a person's chance of experiencing an illness or accident within the upcoming two years based on their stress level. The test is at www.prcn.org/next/stress.html. Take it and see how you do.

Stress triggers are different for each of us. They are a product of our personalities, our relationships, and the circumstances of our life, some of which we can control, much of which is out of our control. The trick is to figure out what we can change and what we cannot change. The only workable response to stress triggers we cannot change is to adapt how we let them make us feel.

The following quiz will help you determine what sets you off.

Your Hot Buttons: A Test

Number each of the following groups of phrases from one to four, with one being the thing that most annoys you and four being the thing that least annoys you or that doesn't bother you at all. When you're done, count your number of As, Bs, Cs, and Ds, then look at the key below to determine your most sensitive hot buttons.

1. a. ___ You're stuck in traffic, and late to work, and you can't find the keys to your filing cabinet where the report you have to present in one hour is tucked away.

   b. ___ You got a poor night's sleep and feel out of sorts.

   c. ___ Your spouse made a negative comment about your new haircut.

   d. ___ You just bought a new power suit, but on the way to work, some yahoo splashed coffee, and now you have to go to your big meeting with a stained collar.

2. a. ___ You suffered through 10 days of 95+ heat with a broken air conditioning unit, and the repairman can't make it to your house for three more days.

  b. ___ You have a nagging cough that never seems to go away.

  c. ___ You heard that your company might merge with a competitor and some jobs will be eliminated.

  d. ___ Your weird neighbor told you your lawn looks nice, and now you are wondering what that was all about.

3. a. ___ There's no way you're going to have your quarterly projections finished by Friday and you know your jerk of a boss will have your hide.

  b. ___ You've hit 40 and no matter what you do, your waistline just keeps expanding.

  c. ___ The possibility of more terrorist attacks.

  d. ___ When your secretary told you the report she was typing was going to be late, you blew up, and now you can't stop blaming yourself for losing control.

4. a. ___ Your roof is leaking, and you don't have the money to fix it, and it keeps getting worse with each rainstorm.

  b. ___ You bought an expensive treadmill, but now you're using it for a clothes hanger, and every time you see it, you feel a stab of guilt.

  c. ___ Your older brother bullies you, and every time you see him, it brings back terrible memories that make you feel small and inadequate, and you just heard he bought the house across the street from you.

  d. ___ Your friends tell you to quit being so hard on yourself, but if they really knew you they'd dislike you, too.

5. a. ___ The chemical plant down the road just blew some kind of noxious gunk into the air.

  b. ___ Your back hurts all the time.

  c. ___ You have a stack of bills and no idea how to pay them.

  d. ___ You wanted to make junior partner by age 30. You're already 29 and nothing seems to be happening and you're panicked that you might be a failure.

6. a. ___ Your new puppy had an accident on your expensive Oriental rug.

  b. ___ You suffer from debilitating migraines almost every day.

  c. ___ Your child is failing algebra and won't study.

  d. ___ You have a blemish the size of a headlight on your chin.

7. a. ___ It's the end of the month, and you've had to work two 60-hour weeks in a row and you're exhausted.

  b. ___ You had an accident, totaled your new car, and hurt your neck.

  c. ___ Your spouse snores, and you can't ever get a decent night's sleep.

      d. ___ You worked so hard to make sure everyone had a great time at the office Christmas party that you wore yourself to a frazzle and couldn't enjoy the party yourself for worrying.

8. a. ___ The weatherman just predicted a hard freeze and your pipes aren't wrapped.

      b. ___ If you have to look at one more chili cheeseburger you'll get sick, but that's all they serve at the only lunch place close to your job.

      c. ___ Your teenager got a tattoo and a nose ring without first discussing it with you.

      d. ___ You can't understand why your spouse gets mad when you pick out their clothes and tell them how to wear their hair. After all, you're just trying to help.

9. a. ___ Even though you're all grown-up, your mother still treats you like a helpless child.

      b. ___ You're going gray and starting to get a few aches and pains.

      c. ___ You gave in to your spouse and bought the big house, but now you're so busy with maintenance and paying bills that you feel overwhelmed.

      d. ___ Your so-called friends complain about your habit of putting yourself down in public.

10. a. ___ When you bought your house there was hardly anyone else in the neighborhood; now it's crowded and noisy.

      b. ___ You can't eat a bite without getting painful heartburn.

      c. ___ A burglar broke into the house next door and you're worried that you might be next.

      d. ___ You just spent two hours printing out a report but noticed a minute smear in the corner of every page. Now you have to start all over again.

Puzzle Key

Mostly A's. You are most sensitive to environmental stresses. You get upset over things like lousy weather, traffic, noise, pollution, big crowds, a cluttered office or home environment, overbooked schedules, long work hours with no relief, and stressful interpersonal relationships with family, friends, and coworkers.

Mostly B's. You are most sensitive to physical stresses. You worry about your health, getting older, gaining weight, what you should eat, getting exposed to illness, how much you do or don't exercise, getting enough sleep, being physically helpless, and possibly getting injured in an accident.

Mostly C's. You are most sensitive to psychological stresses. You are a worrier, always beset with anxiety about one thing or another. You battle with feelings of insecurity and self-esteem, and may find yourself the victim of an office or neighborhood bully. Your emotions make you feel overwhelmed and helpless and sometimes you can't figure out how you will be able to cope with all of life's pressures.

Mostly D's. You are most sensitive to self-generated stress. No matter how well things may be going in your life, you have an internal voice that tells you something is wrong. You are hypercritical of yourself, your appearance, your personality, your abilities all come under merciless fire. From you. You can't accept compliments easily, and think people have some ulterior motive for being nice to you. You're a perfectionist who likes to have things your way and be in total control of every situation.

Mixed results. If you end up with a roughly equal amount of As, Bs, Cs, and Ds, then you are an equal-opportunity worrier who frets over just about everything.

Now that you know what triggers your stress reaction, it's time to figure out what you can do to protect your health by learning how to defuse stressful situations.

You Can Change *Your* World, but Not *the* World

A big part of stress is the feeling of helplessness it engenders. When life is coming at us from every direction and we don't have a plan to deal with it, it's very easy to get overwhelmed and let problems solve themselves by default.

This approach usually leads to more and bigger problems, so why not resolve right now to learn how to meet your stress head on? Develop methods to handle stress that protect both your physical and psychological health and lead to more positive outcomes for everyone involved.

One of the first principles of good stress management is to figure out what you can change. If you skip this important step, you could spend your time like Don Quixote, jousting at windmills and making very little forward progress in your life.

Your thoughts and your actions are definitely within your control. The thoughts and actions of other people are not within your control. You can control the temperature inside your home, but you cannot control the weather outside.

When something worries or upsets you, ask yourself this question: What about this situation is within my control and what is not within my control? Answering these questions will show

Health Notes

The Greek philosopher Epictetus really understood stress management. In 135 B.C.E., he said: "Some things are in our control and others are not." If you can learn what is actually within your control and direct your efforts at change toward that, you'll be a lot happier with your results than if you try to "fix" something that isn't within your power to change.

you very clearly where you can make real changes, and where you must make adaptations within your own thinking because the power to affect change is not within your control.

With this in mind, let's look at the four different types of stressors and see how people who are affected by each one can make some positive steps to improve their stress response.

Calming Your Environment

If you are sensitive to environmental stress, take care to make sure that your work and home environments are clutter-free, well thought out and workable. Choose colors that soothe your senses, and consider purchasing a "white noise" machine if unpleasant noises like barking dogs or construction machinery intrude on your serenity. Burn candles with your favorite scents if you are sensitive to unpleasant odors. Consider the purchase of a small tabletop fountain if you find the sound of running water is calming. If traffic makes you crazy, try to take a job closer to home to eliminate some time from your commute. Better yet, see if your company is amenable to the idea of telecommuters so that you can work from your home. If neither plan is feasible, make sure you have soothing music for your car's CD player to help you cope.

Do everything you can to make your environment nurturing and soothing. It will greatly improve your productivity and reduce the amount of time you spend worrying if your physical space is comforting to you.

Relieving Physical Stress

If you are sensitive to physical stress, get a complete physical to assess your current state of health. If your doctor makes suggestions regarding your diet and exercise, try to follow his advice as best you can (but don't stress over it!). Regular exercise not only improves your cardiovascular health and helps you lose weight, tone up, and gain strength, it also releases endorphins, chemicals that make us feel good. A good diet and regular exercise along with a regular sleep schedule are essential to maintaining your sense of well-being and reducing the amount of time you spending worrying over your body.

Healing Your Mind

If you are sensitive to psychological stress, make a list of the people and situations that trigger your stress. If you are being bullied at work, tell the appropriate person, and if they do not act to relieve the situation, consider changing jobs to get yourself out of the line of fire. If it is your spouse or significant other who is bullying you, consider whether the price you are paying to maintain that relationship is too high. Change as many of the situations that are stressing you as possible to give yourself a feeling of empowerment and control over your situation. When you have done that, assess whatever is not in your control and take steps to change the way you let the situation make you feel. The newfound sense of accomplishment and purpose you gain from taking charge of your life and making positive changes in your circumstances will give you the impetus to take this step.

Letting Go of Self-Generated Stress

If you are sensitive to self-generated stress, it might be a good idea to seek professional assistance to help you get a handle on your habit of worrying. You have to give up the idea that you can control the world through sheer will power and you have to start being kinder to yourself. Everyday, list one thing you like about yourself. Banish negative thoughts. Create a mental flashcard like a big red "Stop!" sign that you automatically bring to the front of your mind whenever you start being hard on yourself. Leave visual cues around your environment to remind you to be nice to yourself. When something happens that embarrasses or upsets you, remember that other people do not experience the situation with quite the same dramatic flair that you do. Keep telling yourself, "I'm okay. I don't have to be perfect." And give yourself a big hug at least once a day. Once you get over your desire to please and control, you might find there are lots of other people who want to hug you everyday, too.

When Fight Is Better Than Flight

There are some situations where you really just don't want to give in to the desire to flee. When an angry spouse or a rebellious child or a dream job with one nasty boss or a heartfelt cause is too important to walk away from, you may desire to stay and duke it out.

There are smart ways and not-so-smart ways to fight. In this section, we'll outline some savvy tips for staying in the ring with the most difficult of opponents, and also tell you about some self-defeating tactics you should avoid.

Fighting Smart

The number one rule of smart fighting is to keep a cool head. Yes, that's easier said than done, but it's not impossible. It takes a bit of thoughtful planning, focus, and commitment. Remember the old saying: "Fight the good fight." What that means is that any fight worth winning is worth fighting well.

We all know people who seem to be itching for a fight all the time. When dealing with people like this, don't play their game. If they are yelling, say gently but firmly, "I can see that you're upset. I'll come back when we can discuss this quietly," and then leave. Don't allow yourself to get drawn into their drama. This technique works well with everyone from spouses to children, friends, and co-workers.

Stay focused on the subject at hand. Don't bring up incidents from past conflicts. If your opponent brings them up, say quietly, "That has no bearing on what we're discussing today," and then steer the conversation back to where it should be.

Offer sincere compliments. If you can show your opponent that you truly appreciate an idea he's had or a thoughtful gesture she made, it will serve to cool the temperature of the fight and refocus attention on the matter at hand.

If your spouse picks at your choice in clothing, why bother asking his opinion? If he says, "I hate that dress you're wearing!" reply simply and quietly, "I'm sorry you feel that way. I like it," and walk away. If he persists, or orders you to take the dress off, don't get drawn into an argument. You're a grown-up and you don't have to offer justification to anyone as to why you like a particular dress, wine, movie, restaurant, or pair of shoes. You just do. Enough said.

It's amazing how many hours we waste arguing over petty things like this. If we all made it our business to respect each other's choices and not harp away when someone does something we don't like, the planet would be a happier place.

Just remember to take turns. If he goes to see your three-hankie tearjerker without making a negative comment, you owe it to him to accompany him to the wrestling match with similar grace. And if you really just cannot stand each other's recreational activities, plan separate outings. The key is to send the other person out the door with a kiss and a heartfelt wish for an enjoyable day. If you send them away crabbing about how they are going off and leaving you on your own, they're going to make you pay when they get back. You don't want that, do you?

If someone is being childish, treating them with respect and courtesy instead of stooping into the fight will eventually put the squelcher on their inappropriate behavior.

Changing Your Expectations

If every single time your mother has visited your house, she's had something nasty to say about your housekeeping, exactly what sort of cosmic event do you think it would take to make her change her behavior? Remember that old "Change what is within your control" thing we keep harping on? Can you control your mother's behavior? Absolutely not. Can you minimize your exposure to her criticism? You sure can. Instead of having her over to your house, take her to a café or out to a movie. If she asks why you aren't taking her to your house anymore, say quietly and without emotion, "I would love to have you over Mom, but you always complain that my house is dirty. So I decided to meet you away from my house from now on."

This kind of quiet explanation is much more likely to get your mother to examine her own behavior and see that it is not conducive to a mature and mutually loving adult relationship. You have a better chance of making a breakthrough using this technique than by standing nose-to-nose with your mother and screaming it out. Big fights usually only send the combatants to their respective corners, bloodied, bruised, but not broken, and still not at all convinced that they themselves played any part in the fight.

Don't Play the Victim

If you're the poor, benighted soul that everyone is always picking on, anyone new you meet is likely to want to jump on the wagon, too. When you wear a sign that says, "Kick me," few people will be able to resist. But why offer up yourself as a victim? Present yourself instead as a capable, confident, and empowered individual who is firmly in charge of their own life, yet open to all of life's many wonderful possibilities. In the same way you learn to ride a bicycle, you can learn to see the glass as half full. Look at Scrooge. Was there ever a more miserable, miserly individual than that old misanthrope? Yet he learned to love life and love his fellow man once again.

Finally, don't allow yourself to get drawn into other topics. That only serves to expand the fight and does nothing to resolve the dispute on the table.

Not-So-Smart-Fighting

These techniques throw fuel on a fire instead of ending conflict:

- Raising your voice
- Making fun of your opponent
- Comparing your opponent unfavorably with a rival
- Making unsubstantiated accusations
- Buying into your opponent's drama
- Trying to draw other people into the conflict to bolster your own position
- Talking about the conflict to others who are not involved

Don't Let the Blankety-Blanks Get You Down

When all is said and done, you are the one who is in charge of how you feel. When you let other people belittle and diminish you, you are giving away some of your power. Whatever you do, don't let people draw you down to their level or into their intrigues. Review the stress management techniques in the next chapter and pick a couple that appeal to you. Practice them until you can easily call on them anytime and anywhere. Then the next time your big lug of a boss screams at you, just close your eyes and take 10 deep breaths, imagine yourself on a Caribbean beach, or whatever works for you. The point is, by taking charge of your own sense of well-being, you have given yourself the tools you need to get out of the line of fire. And that's a very smart move.

The Least You Need to Know

♦ The first step in effective stress management is to figure out exactly what triggers your stress response.

♦ The only thing you can truly change is yourself.

♦ Whether you choose to avoid stress or fight it out, you can protect yourself by handling the situation calmly.

♦ Sometimes the best way to avoid stress is to just get yourself out of the situation.

Chapter 19

Tools and Techniques to Manage Stress

In This Chapter

◆ Considering professional help

◆ Meditate on this

◆ The scent of serenity

◆ The power of prayer

◆ Walking, talking, breathing, rubbing, writing, and laughing it out

◆ When all else fails, medicate

Now that you know what triggers your stress, the next step is to figure out a way to get a handle on it. There are many effective stress management tools—exercise, meditation, counseling, massage, and journaling, among others—and all of them can give you a better sense of empowerment and control over how you feel about the stressful circumstances of your life.

What works best will vary from person to person. Some people like massages and find them relaxing; other people cannot stand to be touched by total strangers. Just remember there is no one "right" answer for stress management. If you try one technique and it doesn't appeal to you, try something else. Discovering what works best for you might take some trial and error, but keep going until you find something you like and that you believe is effective in helping you deal with your stress.

Before you get going, remember, this is supposed to be enjoyable, not grim, so if something you try doesn't make you feel good, just discard it and move on to another idea. Once you discover a stress management technique that works for you, practice it until it becomes second nature. That way, it will always be available for you to call upon instantly when you need stress relief. So go out there, get your game face on, and tackle your stress head-on. This is one contest you *will* win.

When to Get Outside Help

If you feel stuck in one place and the very idea of tackling your stress all by yourself leaves you quaking in your boots, it might be a good idea to seek professional help. A good place to start is the Yellow Pages of your phone book. Just about any major metropolitan area will have several listings under "stress management." Many community colleges offer weekend or night courses in stress management, and you might even find courses offered at the YMCA or by local recreational centers.

If you live in a small community and cannot find any specific listings for stress management in your phone book, call several of the listed psychologists and ask if they know of anyone in the area who specializes in the treatment of stress. If you have access to the Internet and cannot find anyone to help you locally, try entering "stress management" into a search engine to see if you can locate an online support group. Sometimes simply corresponding with people who are facing similar problems can be a big help in dealing with your stress.

The Art of Meditation

Meditation has been practiced for thousands of years in many different cultures. Widely considered to be one of the best stress reduction tools, it's particularly prevalent in Eastern cultures.

One of the earliest tools for meditation was the labyrinth, a self-contained circle or rectangle laid out on the ground or within a garden, where people walked while following a pattern of paths wound intricately within the external shape. Ancient labyrinths have been found on the Grecian island of Crete, as well as in Peru, Egypt, and India. The Hopi Indians of our own North American continent considered the labyrinth to be a sacred symbol of the connection between man and the divine.

Wellness Words

According to the *Merriam-Webster's Dictionary*, **meditate** means to reflect or ponder, to focus one's thoughts, or to engage in contemplation or reflection.

From the beginning, various cultures have held the labyrinth to be sacred or to have magical properties. Scandinavian fishermen walked labyrinths before they launched their nets to ensure a good catch. Other ancient cultures considered life itself to be a labyrinth, and they built labyrinths as physical manifestations of that belief. Most often they were constructed as places of spiritual contemplation. Laid out in a mathematically precise fashion, labyrinths were believed to cure certain ailments and to open walkers up to the possibility of divine communication.

Today, we commonly refer to meditation as a time of quiet contemplation and solitude, a time to pause and reflect, to gather our thoughts, and to calm our hearts.

Ways to Meditate

There are different schools of meditation. Some advise sitting quietly in a yoga pose. Others, including proponents of transcendental meditation, advocate chanting a mantra while meditating to encourage feelings of calmness and spiritual well-being. There is even a modern movement of people who believe in the ancient power of labyrinths; they practice what they call walking meditation. But whatever form you chose, there are some requirements that are constant.

Always meditate in the same place. Chose a quiet place that is free from drafts and neither too hot nor too cold. Make sure the space is open and uncluttered. If you have a low window with a beautiful view, that would make a lovely meditation spot.

Choose Comfortable Clothing

Dress in comfortable clothing, either a unitard or loose top and pants. Leave your feet bare. If they are subject to cold, wear a pair of light cotton socks. If your hair is long, sweep it up and secure it to your head to prevent being distracted by it. Select a comfortable mat or cushion to sit on. If you desire to meditate with candles burning or soft music playing in the background, gather these materials ahead of time.

Choose a comfortable meditation pose. If you are a beginner, do not attempt to twist your body into an uncomfortable or unfamiliar pose just because it is something you have seen in a photograph or drawing. The goal is to select a pose that is relaxing so that the pose itself doesn't interfere with the quality of your meditation.

Finally, decide what sort of meditation you'd like to try. The practice has many variations, with excellent books available detailing each type, but generally speaking, meditation is grouped into two main categories, mindful meditation and focused meditation.

In mindful meditation, you try to open up your awareness so that you may experience the passing parade of sights, sounds, and smells without judging them or forming opinions about them. Mindful meditation sharpens your senses as you learn to take in whatever is happening around you without engaging in any sort of reactive behavior or thoughts.

In focused meditation, you sit quietly and focus your attention on your breath as you breathe in and out. As you develop your skill, you will learn how to slow your breathing and experience a deep sense of tranquility.

Finding Time to Meditate

Now for the difficult part. If you're a parent with small children or have a stressful job, how do you find time to meditate? You have to make it a priority, just as you do with exercise, bill paying, or any other important activity. Schedule meditation time into each day, and do not let anything intrude.

If you're a morning person, get up 15 to 20 minutes earlier than usual and meditate in the quiet of the morning before the rest of the household stirs. If you're a night person, you might like to meditate after everyone else has gone to bed. If you're a mother, you might schedule meditation during your baby's nap. The important thing is to hold the time as something sacred that nothing may intrude upon.

From the Medicine Chest

The physical and mental benefits of meditation have been proven in many studies. When practiced regularly, meditation can:

- Decrease anxiety
- Reduce resting heart rate
- Lower blood pressure
- Decrease levels of serum cortisol, a chemical associated with stress
- Decrease depression
- Increase feeling of vitality
- Increase feeling of empowerment and self-control

All the more reason to start meditating now!

It will take you a little time to get the hang of it, but as with anything else that takes a bit of practice to perfect, you will soon find meditating as natural as breathing.

A Good Scent Soothes the Soul

Aromatherapy is as ancient a practice as meditation. For thousands of years, aromatic plants and their essential oils were used for a variety of medicinal purposes by everyone from the ancient Egyptians to the Greeks, Romans, Chinese, and even the Aztecs. With the exception of smelling salts, a strong combination of odors used to arouse someone who has fainted, the art of aromatherapy was lost to modern man. Happily, a revival was launched a few years ago, and now aromatherapy products are available almost every-where.

There are now several good aromatherapy products on the market that contain combinations of oils designed specifically for stress relief. You can choose from candles, potpourri, sleep pillows, sachets, massage or bath oils, room sprays, and a variety of bath products. Select a scent that is soothing to you and buy a range of products in that scent.

Aromatherapy for Stress Relief

While essential oils have been used effectively for many medicinal purposes, we will focus on oils proven useful for the purposes of stress relief. Please note that all the following oils also have other medicinal and healing uses not listed here. Only their stress-related benefits are given.

- ◆ **Lavender.** Soothing, calming, balancing, mood lifter, also has antiseptic, analgesic, and antimicrobial properties. Lavender relieves tension, helps to ease depression, and offers excellent relief from stress headaches. Also promotes natural sleep.

 Health Notes _____

When elderly patients in a British nursing home complained of sleep difficulties, not even sleeping pills proved very effective. But when Dr. David Stretch, a researcher at the University of Leicester, wafted the gentle scent of lavender under their noses, all fell asleep quickly and slept soundly. Dried lavender blossoms, one of the most effective scents for promoting sleep, is the primary ingredient in the sleep-inducing pillows that have recently become so popular.

- ◆ **Geranium.** Relaxing, healing, energizing, and can help to soothe a mild headache.
- ◆ **Ylang ylang.** Has a sedative and anti-depressive effect. It also lifts negative moods and calms nervous tension.
- ◆ **Sandalwood.** Relieves tension, stress, depression, and exhaustion. Has a sedative effect.
- ◆ **Jasmine.** Relieves nervous exhaustion, lifts the spirits.
- ◆ **Rosemary.** Beneficial to calm stress and relieve nervousness.
- ◆ **Bergamot.** Relieves tiredness, irritability, and stress. Also used to treat depression.
- ◆ **Chamomile.** Helps to relieve sleeplessness and stress. Known for its calming properties.
- ◆ **Yarrow.** Used to calm nerves, and treat insomnia and stress. Mild sedative.
- ◆ **Clary sage.** Helpful for nervous tension and stress-related disorders. May help soothe headaches.

Using Essential Oils

There are many effective ways to use essential oils to manage stress. The easiest is to buy a simple plastic spray bottle, fill it with filtered water, and add a few drops of your favorite oil to the bottle. Shake it several times and then spray lightly into the air to pleasantly scent a room. Spray your pillow and bedclothes just before retiring to help you drift off to sleep.

Keep a handkerchief with a few drops of your favorite scent in your purse or pocket. Whenever you feel stressed, take it out, hold it up to your nose, and inhale deeply several times. You'll be surprised what a calming and soothing effect this has.

You can also light aromatherapy candles or pour a few drops of essential oil into a specially designed aromatherapy burner.

Relax in a warm tub scented with your favorite oil or add some to a base oil to use for massage. Just before retiring, massage a bit of the scented oil into your temples for a calming effect.

As soothing as these oils can be, don't assume that all essential oils are safe for use in aromatherapy and stress relief just because they're natural. Many oils contain powerful caustic elements that can burn the skin or irritate breathing passages. Here are a few to avoid:

- **Camphor.** May irritate sensitive skin. White camphor is less irritating than other varieties and is the one recommended for use in breathing remedies.

- **Ginger, orange, lemon, or lime.** If applied full strength to the skin, these oils cause discoloration upon exposure to sunlight. The stain will slowly disappear but cannot be removed by scrubbing.

- **Cassia.** The sweet, cinnamon-like smell of this oil disguises the fact that it is a highly reactive skin irritant and poisonous if swallowed.

- **Wintergreen.** A highly toxic oil that should never be put on the skin.

- **Cinnamon.** You won't forget the large red stinging welts you'll get if you put cinnamon oil on your skin. Try the less-reactive cinnamon leaf oil, though even this milder version is not recommended for people with sensitive skin.

- **Pennyroyal.** Despite its folk use as an insect repellant, pennyroyal is a deadly poison and liver toxin that should never be used without the advise of a health-care professional.

- **Clove.** Delicious in cooking but highly irritating to skin and mucous membranes if used in aromatherapy.

A Higher Power

Many people gather comfort from the power of prayer. Whatever your religious beliefs, pausing for a time of quiet prayer can have a soothing and rejuvenating effect, particularly during times of stress.

Prayer can also be a form of meditation. You may wish to consecrate a quiet corner of your home for prayer, or you could create a small altar that contains symbols of your faith. Fire has always been associated with religious ceremony, and you may find it meaningful to light a small candle whenever you pray.

Instead of praying just when you feel stressed, try to develop the habit of praying regularly. The ritual of prayer can become a significant source of stress relief if you make it a regular part of your day-to-day life.

Get Up and Move

Exercise is one of the best stress-busters around. Prolonged aerobic exercise of sufficient duration (at least 30 minutes) releases powerful chemicals called endorphins into your bloodstream. Endorphins produce feelings of euphoria and well-being and are responsible for the well-known "runner's high" that many joggers experience after a long run.

If job stress is threatening to overwhelm you, consider using your lunch break to exercise. Even if you only get a half hour, you can walk for 15 minutes and then grab a sandwich or a smoothie. Very shortly after starting this stress management technique, you will find yourself much more able to cope with whatever stressful situations you encounter. The added bonus is that incorporating regular exercise into your daily routine will almost certainly whittle a few inches from your waistline. (If you need some tips on how to choose the right exercise for you or how to stick to an exercise routine, you can reread Part 3.)

Reach Out and Call Someone

Life's problems always seem more difficult when you try to tackle them by yourself. It helps to talk over problems with sympathetic listeners, but unless you let them know you need help, those closest to you might not know what to do. If you're feeling stressed out, particularly if you're facing a difficult time like the illness of a family member or the loss of a job, don't forget to reach out to your friends. Talking to others can really help you get a handle on stressful situations.

People genuinely want to help their friends who are having difficulties but often do not know how or where to start. If you clearly tell your friends and family members what it is you need from them, you might be surprised what a strong support network they will offer just when you need it most. You can get by much more easily with a little assistance from the people who care for you. All you have to do is ask for their help.

Take Ten Deep Breaths

One of the simplest, quickest, and most effective ways to handle stress is to simply sit down, focus your attention on your breathing, and take 10, deep, full breaths. Keeping your spine erect, inhale through your nose until your lungs are fully inflated. Blow the air slowly out of your mouth until your lungs are completely deflated. For an extra measure of calmness, hold the breath for a count of five before releasing. As you breathe, picture soothing, pleasurable images in your mind—a beautiful beach at sunset, a waterfall, a purring kitten—whatever makes you feel happy. Consciously relax the muscles of your face, neck, and shoulders. Within 10 minutes you will feel completely renewed and much less stressed.

Getting Rubbed the Right Way

Massage therapy is another highly effective method to deal with stress. Many licensed masseuses now regularly visit businesses and office buildings with their portable massage chairs to offer affordable 15-minute stressbuster massages that concentrate on the neck and shoulders—where many of us hold most of our tension. The nice thing is that you can have them right in the office and you don't need to remove your clothing.

From the Medicine Chest

Try the on-the-spot stress relief benefits of acupressure. To relieve headache and eyestrain, use your middle finger to apply steady pressure to the indentation between the top of your nose and the beginning of your forehead. Take slow, deep breaths as you press, then release after one minute. Relax, focus, and repeat. You will be amazed at the quick results.

If you have more time and feel totally stressed out, consider getting a full-body massage. Many salons and day spas now offer massages, along with other relaxing body treatments like Vichy showers, salt rubs, seaweed wraps, and mineralized mud baths.

Massage has many benefits for stress relief. It relieves muscular tension, stiffness, and aches along with any associated discomfort, and it reduces anxiety and improves circulation of both blood and lymph fluid. The next time you're stressed out, try a 15-minute massage and see if that helps you to feel calmer.

Is Laughter the Best Medicine?

Researchers at California's Loma Linda University Medical Center set out to prove whether or not laughter was truly beneficial. They gathered two groups of volunteers. One was shown an hour's worth of funny videos while the control group was seated in a soundproof room. They took blood samples before, during, and after the experiment from both groups.

The results shouldn't surprise anyone who enjoys a good laugh. Volunteers exposed to the comic tapes had increased levels of endorphins and neurotransmitters associated with pleasure circulating in their blood and reduced levels of the stress-related chemicals, cortisol, and adrenaline.

So there you have it, scientific proof that laughter is an effective tool to counter stress. The key is to give yourself permission to laugh, whenever and wherever you are. Remember that famous scene in *Mary Poppins* where everyone laughed so hard they floated up to the ceiling? Laughter is like that; it can make you so happy that you feel light as air and ready to float away. And that's much more pleasant than feeling like you want to slug someone.

Children laugh an average of 400 times a day. By the time we reach adulthood, we laugh an average of just 15 times a day. There's no need to become a sourpuss just because the years are rolling by. Find something that makes you laugh and latch onto it. It could be a silly picture, your favorite joke, a funny scene from a movie, or whatever tickles your funnybone. When you feel stress starting to overwhelm you, get out your "tickler" and laugh until you feel better. It works.

Journal Your Feelings

Some people feel stressed because they don't feel heard. To be heard is to receive validation, but it may not always be possible to get external validation. For example, a single mom with two small children who works a dead-end job at a lunch counter doesn't exactly get too many chances during the course of her day to hear compliments or discuss ideas. But what if this waitress or anyone in a similar situation started a journal and wrote down her most important thoughts and ideas each evening before bed? Then she will have given herself an excellent outlet for managing stress.

Journaling is an excellent tool that helps relieve stress by giving people a tool to feel validated and a way to organize their thoughts. The discipline of journaling imposes a sort of serenity on the writer. If you know that no matter how badly your day has gone you will have 15 minutes before bed to write down all your thoughts and feelings, that knowledge acts as a pressure relief valve and gives you something to look forward to at the end of the day. Extra bonus: If you're a good writer, at the end of a year you might have a saleable manuscript. At the very least, you will have a reliable way to express your feelings safely, and that's one of the best stress-relief tools you will find.

When You Need Medication

If you've tried everything else and stress still rules and ruins your life, you might need to take a prescription medication for a while to get you through the rough patch. Start with your family physician and see if he or she can prescribe a mild sedative to help you relax.

If you're having trouble sleeping, ask if there is something you can take for a short while (two weeks or less at most) that will help you get the rest you need. Remember that unrelenting stress can lead to a host of other health problems, so don't be afraid to ask for medical help to manage your stress and keep it from evolving into something more dangerous.

The Least You Need to Know

◆ There are many effective techniques to manage stress.

◆ Try several different techniques to see what works best for you.

◆ Try combining different therapies for maximum benefit.

◆ Don't be afraid to seek professional help or ask for medication if you can't manage your stress on your own.

20

To Sleep, Perchance to Dream

In This Chapter

- ◆ Why we need sleep
- ◆ How sleep disturbances cause stress
- ◆ The dangers of sleep deprivation
- ◆ Tips for a good night's sleep
- ◆ Sleep disorders

Perhaps the most famous insomniac in the world was Hamlet, who roamed the ramparts of his stepfather's castle each midnight, lamenting the foibles of his dysfunctional family. You may not have ramparts to roam, but chances are if you have trouble sleeping, you may have a well-worn patch of carpet or favorite easy chair where you try to work out your sleeplessness. Family problems are but one of many reasons sleep may be disturbed. Financial worries, job problems, aging, an impending big event like a marriage or the birth of a child, or physical illness including heartburn, indigestion, and pain can all contribute to difficulty in sleeping.

So what's the big deal if you lose a few winks? If it's an occasional occurrence related to an easily identified temporary situation, it's not so serious. However, if trouble getting to sleep or staying asleep is an ongoing difficulty, you could be heading for real health problems.

In this chapter, we'll take a look at the many facets of sleep—how to get to sleep, how to stay asleep, and things you can do to make sure you wake up refreshed. We also review the most common causes of sleep disturbance and how to resolve them.

Why Is Sleep Necessary?

In modern America, a society that fires on all cylinders 24/7, we have come to almost resent the very idea of going to sleep. We think of sleeping as "wasted hours" and keep trying to figure out how to get by on less and less sleep.

No idea could be more wrongheaded. Sleep is one of the most important activities of the day in terms of maintaining wellness, because it is during sleep that the body repairs itself and the mind and spirit are renewed. During the day you burn off energy as you move through your day's activities; while you sleep those energy stores are replenished. During the day you might sustain minor injuries, small tears in your muscles or scrapes or cuts on your skin; during the night your body repairs itself. During the day you may deal with numerous stressful situations at work or at home; a good night's sleep helps you to awaken mentally refreshed and ready to tackle problems anew.

Uninterrupted sleep is necessary so the body can cycle through all the stages of sleep, including the deepest level of sleep, Rapid Eye Movement sleep, or REM, the dream state, which is the most restorative and necessary sleep phase for the body.

 Health Notes

Napoleon Bonaparte was a famous insomniac. Here's one of his lesser-known quotes regarding the necessity for sleep: "Six hours of sleep are adequate for a man, seven for a woman, and eight for a fool."

In short, a good night's sleep is one of the best ways to ensure your continued good health, while ongoing sleep disturbances are one of the fastest routes to illness. So if you're reading this book at midnight, put it down, fluff up your pillows, lie down, close your eyes, and go to sleep. That's an order. You can finish this chapter tomorrow when you're feeling rested.

Which Comes First—the Stress or the Sleeplessness?

Stress and sleeplessness form a conundrum—sleeplessness causes stress, but stress is one of the most frequent causes of sleeplessness. So which comes first?

Stress is the initial culprit. We've all had nights when sleep just wouldn't come, nights when we've had a fight with a spouse or a friend or were worried about paying a house note on time or losing our jobs. As we tossed and turned, replaying the troubling event over and over again in our minds, our pulse and blood pressure steadily increased along with our body temperature, and sleep slipped farther and farther away.

Stress increases the amount of cortisol circulating in our bloodstreams. In addition to the physical effects just mentioned, cortisol also stimulates increased production of gastric acid, which can cause bedtime heartburn and acid indigestion, only adding to the sleep problem.

If stress is causing your sleeplessness, try some of the stress management techniques outlined in Chapter 19, "Tools and Techniques to Manage Stress." If the problem goes deeper than that, keep reading to see if you might be suffering from a sleep disorder.

Six to Eight Hours a Night

We live in a busy, hectic world, and we all try to cram way too many activities into a single day. The first thing that suffers when we overbook our schedules is sleep. We tell ourselves we can get by with three or four hours and keep right on going, but sleep deprivation is cumulative. Each time you cheat yourself out of an hour or two of sleep, you add to your *sleep deficit* tab. So if you have one late night in the course of a week and miss a couple of hours of sleep, it will be easy enough to make it up by sleeping an extra hour on Saturday and Sunday mornings. But if you miss 3 hours of sleep every weekday night, you'll build up a sleep deficit of 15 hours by Saturday, and that's an awful lot to make up in one weekend.

Of course, we all have different sleep personalities. Some of us rise with the dawn and droop with the sunset, while others don't really perk up until mid-morning and can stay up half the night without blinking an eye. And some of us get grumpy if we get less than eight hours of sleep every night, while others do fine with just six or seven.

"I don't need much sleep," you may be telling yourself. Oh, but you do. Our bodies were designed to function optimally with a full six to eight hours of rest each night, and when we get less, things start going haywire.

Wellness Words

Sleep deficit is the difference between the number of hours of sleep you need—about six to eight—and the number of hours you actually get. For example, if you get just 4 hours of sleep per night all week long, by Saturday you'd have a 20-hour sleep deficit for that week.

A Fast Track to Aging

For starters, people who skimp on sleep age faster. Yes, they *age faster*, and it's been proven scientifically. The same study showed that chronic sleep deprivation greatly increases the odds of developing health problems, including diabetes, high blood pressure, obesity, and memory loss. That's a pretty steep price to pay just to run an extra load of laundry or balance you checkbook late at night.

Endocrinologists at the University of Chicago conducted a study, published in the August 16, 2000, issue of the *Journal of the American Medical Association*, and found evidence of accelerated aging in 11 otherwise healthy young men in their 20s less than one week after they were limited to just 4 hours of sleep per night for the study. The test subjects were affected in several ways. After being subjected to the nightly sleep deprivation, the subjects' glucose tolerance tested at levels typical of men in their 60s. They all started releasing more of the stress hormone cortisol during the day at rates that were typical of middle-aged adults, not healthy young males.

Because lack of sleep causes your body to release more cortisol, that's a clear indication you will feel more stressed after you've slept poorly or for too few hours. When you go several nights without getting enough sleep, the effects of stress will continue to multiply and accumulate. Long-term overexposure to cortisol can lead to a number of serious health problems, including hardening of the arteries, stomach ulcers, headaches, higher cholesterol, hypertension, a greater tendency toward blood clots, lower immunity to infections, greater susceptibility to asthma, and emotional or behavioral disorders.

You can save yourself from many of these health problems simply by developing good sleep habits and sticking to them. Making sure you get eight full hours of restful sleep each night is a very good way to support both your mental and physical health.

Sleep Deprivation Is Dangerous

Sleep deprivation is not just a health issue; it can be downright dangerous. A lack of sleep does more than make you feel sleepy. It can contribute to accidents and derail your coping skills. Minor disagreements may escalate to all-out war if the combatants are both sleep-deprived. Sleep deprivation can also cause more immediate and readily apparent effects:

- Irritability and crankiness
- Decreased cognitive ability
- Decreased coordination
- Impaired judgment and analytical ability
- Slower reaction time

> **CAUTION**
>
> **911!**
>
> Don't drive if you are sleep-deprived. According to the National Highway Traffic Safety Administration, sleep deprivation causes more than 100,000 motor vehicle accidents annually, with 1,500 fatalities. If you're driving and start to feel sleepy, pull over and stop immediately. Take a 20- or 30-minute catnap and only start driving again when you feel alert. It may save your life.

You can imagine that if you're showing up at work each day displaying any of these symptoms listed, your job performance is going to suffer. All the more reason to make sure you get a good night's sleep every night.

Researchers are also beginning to take a hard look at the role fatigue and sleep deprivation play in accidents and workplace safety. The National Highway Traffic Safety
Commission says driver fatigue is the major contributing factor in 30 to 40 percent of all
crashes involving 18-wheelers each year. Cross-country truckers, famous for going on a
few winks and a cup of joe, might take the time to get enough sleep if they realized their
bravado was costing so many lives.

It's Not Just Car Crashes

Lack of adequate sleep has been cited as a contributing factor in several plane crashes
when pilot fatigue led to errors in judgment that caused a loss of control of the aircraft.
Investigations of accidents with heavy machinery often show the operator was working
without adequate rest. Medication errors in hospitals happen more frequently when
interns and nurses are fatigued. Government investigators listed sleep deprivation as one
of the main reasons for the *Challenger* disaster. Maintenance crews responsible for check-
ing the O-rings on the shuttle were going on so little sleep they were practically cross-
eyed.

Chernobyl, Three-Mile Island, the *Exxon Valdez*—reports on all of these disasters lay
some blame on the extreme fatigue of key decision-making personnel. If you work in a
critical job and feel forced to keep going around the clock, perhaps you should show your
boss some statistics on sleep-related accidents. If you slow down and get enough sleep, not
only will you arrive at work feeling more energized and enthusiastic, but your productivity
will soar. It's been proven in study after study, and that's news that should make any boss
happy.

According to the National Sleep Foundation, sleepy workers cost U.S. employers more
than $18 billion annually in lost productivity. That figure zooms even higher when you
add in the cost of fatigue-related accidents and errors and consequent health claims.
When the organization conducted a survey of American workers, 51 percent said that
sleepiness on the job impairs their productivity. Sixty-eight percent admitted they had
problems getting enough sleep. The National Sleep Foundation estimates that at any
given time, 64 percent of Americans are working in a state of sleep deprivation.

Good Habits Make for Good Sleep

Despite its name, sleep hygiene has nothing to do with cleanliness and everything to do
with routine and dependability. By routine, we mean following a bedtime ritual that signals your body and brain that it is time for sleep. By dependability, we mean going to
sleep at roughly the same time every night so your brain and body can depend on that
time.

Wellness Words

Circadian rhythms are cycles of biological activity and behavior that occur generally within a 24-hour period that are generated by an internal clock synchronized to light-dark cycles in the environment.

Before the invention of the electric light bulb, people had no choice. When it got dark, they had to wind down or face a fortune in candle bills. When we lived that way, we were closer to our biological roots than now, when the world is ablaze in a wash of neon color 24 hours a day. Still, lights or no lights, as biological beings we are subject to the same *circadian rhythms* that govern all of nature.

And you know what they say about not messing with Mother Nature. Good advice aside, many of us do mess with Mother Nature anyway, going to sleep at 2 A.M. one night, dropping like a sack of lead into bed at 8:30 P.M. the next, and then staying up until midnight the next. One night we dose off in the recliner, the next night we fall asleep next to our cranky child on a narrow bunk bed, and the next night we're on the sofa because our spouse is snoring. It's no wonder our poor bodies and brains don't know what to do, and it's no wonder our sleep cycles get all messed up.

To encourage restful slumber, you need to establish a few good bedtime habits, or good sleep hygiene as it is called in the world of sleep disorders.

1. Get at least six to eight hours of sleep per night.

2. Keep regular sleep habits. Go to bed within a half hour of the same time each evening, and wake up at about the same time each morning. This helps to "set" your body's biological clock and teaches your body to expect sleep at a certain time every day.

3. If you're on a regular 9-to-5 schedule, make sure to go to bed before midnight. Your body's natural rhythms make you feel sleepier then. After midnight, you may get a second surge of energy and alertness that will make it difficult for you to fall asleep.

4. Regular exercise helps people to sleep better, but don't exercise just before bed because it may disrupt your sleep. Aim for the morning or late afternoon.

5. Don't allow yourself to nap while reading or watching television. Even a short nap can interfere with your ability to fall asleep later that evening.

6. Avoid stimulants such as coffee, nicotine, tea, colas, chocolate, and certain prescription or over-the-counter drugs that contain caffeine in the late afternoon and evening hours. They can make it more difficult for you to fall asleep, particularly if you are already feeling stressed.

7. Don't eat a large meal too close to bedtime, particularly if the menu contains spicy foods. Heartburn and indigestion are two of the most frequent causes of insomnia.

8. Don't drink a large amount of fluid before going to bed, or you'll find yourself getting up in the middle of the night to urinate.

9. Taking a drink or two may help a person fall asleep more quickly, but it disrupts sleep patterns later in the night. You may experience nightmares, severe headaches, or other undesirable side effects as a result of excessive alcohol consumption near bedtime.

10. Keep your bed for sleeping. Read in a comfortable chair, not in bed, and confine your work to a desk or office area. Food should stay in the kitchen or dining area. If you associate your bed only with sleep (and of course, romance), it is more likely you will fall asleep quickly once you get in bed.

11. Don't watch the clock. If you are having trouble falling asleep, the worst thing you can do is keep looking at the time. Put the clock in a place where you cannot see it from your bed.

If you've followed all these suggestions and are still having trouble falling asleep, pay a little attention to your sleep environment. Are your mattress, pillows, and bedding comfortable? Do you need a fan? A night light? Is your bed in a convenient spot? Is the room too cool? Too hot? Is it quiet? Determine what it is you need to make yourself feel comfortable in your sleep environment and then provide it. If you travel a lot, bring along a favorite pillow or something else that will feel comfortable and familiar, to encourage sleep.

But I'm Too Worried to Sleep

If you're one of those people who feel like you just can't turn off your mind at bedtime, whose thoughts race madly like mice in a maze, then you should schedule some "worry" time in the early evening. Put a small trash can at your bedroom door so you can leave your worries there at night. Write down everything that is bothering you on a sheet of paper. Discuss it with your spouse, friend, or anyone else who can serve as your sounding board. Make plans, develop potential solutions, scream, cry, yell, throw things—do whatever you have to do to work out the nervous energy you have tied up in your worries. When it's time for bed, pick up the paper of all your worries and toss it into the trash can at your bedroom door. You can get it back the next morning if you really want to, but for the moment, when you're trying to get to sleep, you don't want those worries anywhere around you. It may take you a few nights to get the hang of this technique, but you'll be surprised at how effective and easy it is to simply write down your worries and then toss them.

Sleep Inducers

There are a number of tricks you can play on yourself to help sleep along. A light bedtime snack of skim milk or other dairy products containing the sleep-promoting amino acid tryptophan can actually help you fall asleep faster.

A warm bath (not a shower) a half-hour before you turn in can work wonders, particularly if you scent the water with a calming, soothing oil like lavender or jasmine. Soft music may also help. You might also want to purchase a unit that combines gentle white noise like waves on a beach with aromatherapy. Several companies now offer pillow sprays containing calming essential oils. Spritz your pillow and bed linens lightly before you lie down, and you'll drift off to sleep enveloped in a blanket of calming lavender.

When It's Time to See a Doctor

Sometimes, no matter what you do or how hard you try, you simply cannot fix your own sleep problems. First, speak to your regular physician whenever sleep becomes a problem for you. As discussed, a physical illness may be at the root of the problem. In any case, your primary physician certainly can aid you as you search for a solution. At some point, you and your doctor may decide that it's time to consult a physician who specializes in sleep disorders.

Sleep specialists are usually neurologists who have undergone additional training. They will take your health history, ask if you feel you have any particular emotional or physical problems, and then take a complete physical. Once the sleep specialist has an idea about the nature of your complaint, he will most likely schedule a sleep study.

Ten years ago, sleep study centers were virtually unheard of in this country. The only ones available were attached to large university research centers or teaching hospitals. Today, almost every major metropolitan hospital has a sleep study center.

When a patient is referred to a sleep lab doctors will conduct an overnight study of their sleeping habits. The patient sleeps in a special sleep center bedroom furnished with the comforts of a typical home plus lots of diagnostic and monitoring equipment. Technicians attach electrodes to the patient's head, chest, and legs in a way that will not interfere with his sleep, and the patient is then hooked up to an EEG to monitor brain waves and an EKG machine to monitor heart activity during the night. The leg electrodes detect muscle tone and leg movement.

Thermisters by the patient's nose and mouth measure respiratory function, and a snore monitor measures vibrations of the throat. The oxygen saturation of the patient's blood is monitored and recorded, as are episodes of snoring and apnea. Pressure transducers strapped around the chest and abdomen measure how hard a person is trying to breathe. A CO_2 monitor near the nose measures the presence of carbon dioxide in air exhaled by the patient. Finally, a video camera enables technicians to see and hear the patient without disturbing his sleep.

You might think it would be impossible to sleep with all that stuff attached to your body, but during sleep center studies, patients generally sleep exactly as they have been sleeping at home, giving doctors a very good idea of their particular difficulty. Following the sleep center tests, the attending specialist makes a diagnosis and refers the patient back to his own doctor with a treatment plan.

Here are some of the most common sleep disorders, along with their symptoms and available treatments.

Insomnia

The dictionary definition of insomnia is the prolonged and usually abnormal inability to obtain adequate sleep. Doctors define insomnia as poor-quality sleep. Whether that occurs because the person has difficulty falling asleep, awakens frequently during the night, awakens too early, or awakens feeling fatigued is not the issue. The issue is that for whatever reason, the quality of sleep insomniacs do get is not refreshing and restoring to them. Chronic insomnia requires medical intervention for successful resolution.

Treatment—Treatment depends on whether the insomnia is transient, intermittent, or chronic. Transient insomnia, related to a specific reason or event, usually resolves itself over a short period of time, perhaps with the use of a sleep medication through the most difficult period. Transient insomnia occurs when something traumatic has occurred, like a death, an accident, or loss of a job, or may be triggered by jet lag.

Intermittent insomnia comes and goes and is related to recurring periods of stress or something in the sleep environment, like a dog barking, that occasionally disturbs the sleeper. Treatment may include temporary use of sleep aides and a change in sleep hygiene to address the cause of the wakefulness.

Chronic insomnia lasts for a month or more and happens almost every night. It may be caused by an underlying psychological condition like depression or the inappropriate use of caffeine or alcohol and is often a problem for people whose sleep and waking patterns are disrupted by their work schedule.

Stress plays a big role in chronic insomnia. One of the most frequent reasons people cite for wakefulness is that once they've had a few bad nights, they start worrying that every night is going to be bad and that worry itself keeps them awake.

If insomnia is making you sleepy during the day and impairing your judgment and performance, your doctor may prescribe a short course of sleeping pills to get you back on track. Counseling may also be helpful if a psychological condition is the underlying cause.

Sleep Apnea

Sleep apnea is a condition in which people stop breathing repeatedly during the course of the night, perhaps hundreds of times, with each episode lasting for as short as a second or two or as long as a minute. It is characterized by abnormally loud snoring punctuated by gasping as the brain signals the body to start breathing again. Victims become progressively more fatigued if they continue without treatment. According to the National Institutes of Health, more than 12 million Americans suffer from sleep apnea with most of the victims being male, significantly overweight, and past the age of 40. Untreated, sleep apnea leads to progressively more serious fatigue and daytime grogginess, and may trigger high blood pressure, heart attack, or stroke.

Treatment—Includes weight reduction programs and CPAP or Continuous Positive Airway Pressure administered through a mask the patient wears while sleeping. The steady stream of pressurized air prevents soft tissue in your throat from collapsing and blocking the breathing passage. If all else fails, your doctor may perform surgery to remove excess soft tissue at the back of your throat.

Restless Leg Syndrome

Restless leg syndrome (RLS) causes involuntary jerking of the legs during the night, interfering with the quality of sleep. It is characterized by itchy, creeping sensations deep within the legs that cause an irresistible urge to move the legs. Movement does temporarily relieve the unpleasant sensations. Doctors are not sure what causes it, but the problem does seem to run in families.

Treatment—Doctors generally start treatment with vitamin therapy, including iron, B-12, and folate. Avoidance of caffeine and alcohol is also helpful. Some drugs prescribed for other conditions, like calcium channel blockers, seem to make the symptoms of RLS worse. Specialists usually prescribe regular moderate exercise and stretching to provide relief. If all else fails, drugs may be prescribed to help control RLS.

Sleepwalking

Also called somnambulism, sleepwalking is one of the most complex of sleep disorders. Normally, the brain manufactures a chemical that paralyzes the body during REM sleep, so your brain can act out dreams without triggering any physical movement. Sleepwalkers lack this chemical, so they get out of bed and act out their dreams. Episodes can last from a few seconds to a half hour or longer and involve simple activities like sitting up to complex tasks like driving a car, all performed while sound asleep. About 18 percent of the population sleepwalks. It's more common in children and in males. The average frequency is one episode per month, but the severe form occurs almost nightly and presents a real risk of physical injury to the sleepwalker.

Treatment—Bedtime regularity is particularly important in treating sleepwalking, as overtiredness can trigger episodes. Stress is also a factor, so a calming program of meditation or deep breathing immediately prior to bedtime can be helpful. Drugs and hypnosis have both proven effective in reducing or eliminating sleepwalking episodes. Until the problem is brought under control, the bedroom should be made as safe as possible. Remove low furniture that could present a tripping hazard, lock windows, particularly in second floor bedrooms, and consider putting an alarm on a sleepwalker's bedroom door to alert you when an episode is underway.

Narcolepsy

Narcolepsy is a neurological sleep disorder characterized by sudden "sleep attacks" in which the victim unexpectedly falls sound asleep in the middle of the day (also called EDS or excessive daytime sleepiness), or suffers an attack of cataplexy, or complete loss of voluntary muscle control.

Treatment—EDS is treated with stimulants that limit daytime sleepiness while cataplexy is treated with anti-depressants and serotonin re-uptake inhibitors. Nap therapy, two to three short naps daily, is also helpful in controlling daytime sleepiness and maintaining alertness. Narcolepsy involves complex social and safety issues that can best be addressed by joining a support group with other sufferers and their families.

Other less common sleep disorders include night terrors and tooth grinding or bruxism. If something is disturbing your sleep on a regular basis, consult your doctor for advice.

The Least You Need to Know

- ◆ A good night's sleep is one of the most essential components of the wellness lifestyle.
- ◆ Loss of sleep causes stress, but stress is one of the most significant causes of loss of sleep.
- ◆ Sleep deprivation contributes to thousands of accidents and fatalities each year.
- ◆ Going to bed at the same time every night promotes a good night's sleep.
- ◆ Sleep disorders require medical intervention.

Part 5

The Fourth Pillar—Preventive Maintenance

Preventive maintenance is the one facet of wellness that all too many people overlook. But incorporating it into your life is one of the smartest things you can do. Learning which signs and symptoms to watch for can help you catch and treat many health problems in the early and more readily managed stages. Following recommendations for annual checkups and exams is another great way to stop small problems before they get out of hand.

In this part, we provide age and gender appropriate checkups you should schedule as a regular part of your wellness program. We also review some of the most common symptoms to look for and what they may mean.

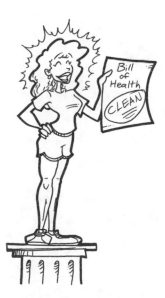

Chapter 21

Checkups to Check Out

In This Chapter

- Who needs a checkup?
- The annual physical
- For women only
- For men only

You are eating right, exercising, getting enough sleep, drinking your water, and you feel fine, so why would you want to go to the doctor? Going to the doctor is for sick people, and you feel great!

There are quite a number of health problems that are without symptoms until they begin to cause problems, such as high blood pressure, diabetes, and glaucoma, so a checkup is a good first step to staying healthy.

It should make sense that you don't want to wait until a small problem becomes a big problem. Your health history or family history might put you in a high-risk category, so getting that checkup can be an important part of staying well.

The Checkup Experts

The U.S. Preventive Services Task Force is an independent panel of experts in primary care and prevention that systematically reviews the evidence of effectiveness of screening tests and other examinations and develops guideline recommendations for preventive services, such as how often you should see your family physician and what for.

From the Medicine Chest

Elevated blood cholesterol is one of the major risk factors for coronary heart disease, the leading cause of death in the United States. It can be modified by diet and medication, but you need to learn if yours is high by getting a blood test.

Breast cancer is the most common form of cancer in women, accounting for 46,000 deaths a year. Check your breasts monthly. Breast cancer is treatable if caught early.

Tobacco use causes one of every five deaths in the United States each year, making it the most important preventable cause of premature death. Smoking-cessation programs and medication can save your life. Talk to your doctor about quitting.

Your Medical History

If the primary care physician you choose to perform these tests has never examined you before, he or she will want to know quite a few things about you. You'll have a lot of answers to give, beginning with general information such as your age, sex, what you do for a living, whether or not you have a significant other, and who he should call in case you need to go to the hospital.

You should list as much information as you can recall about any previous illnesses, hospitalizations, or accidents you have had, as well as any specific problems that run in your family. Let your doctor know about recent weight loss, any trouble you have sleeping, and any aches, pains, depression, or unusual fatigue.

There are lots of things you can tell him that will help with a diagnosis. This isn't a game where you make the doctor try to guess about what might be wrong with you, if anything. This is a time when you want to give him as much information as possible about you and your lifestyle.

If you smoke or regularly drink, tell the doctor. The doctor will want to know details of your work and leisure. If you operate lawn mower, your doctor may better understand any hearing loss. If you jump in and out of a delivery truck many times a day, that may point to a possible explanation of your recurrent knee injury. Your bad golf swing could explain the pain in your hip. Your loud snoring could be an indication of sleep apnea, a dangerous condition that could result in death.

This is your chance to whine about anything and everything to someone who is willing to listen, even though he or she is getting paid to do it. Something you don't think is important may send the physician in the right direction to discover why your stomach hurts all the time. It might not be an ulcer that you secretly suspect and worry that you have; it may be caused by the aspirin you take right before bed to stop the pain in your lower back.

Before your appointment ...

1. Make a list of things you would like to talk to the doctor about. How many times have you complained after you leave the doctor's office that you forgot to ask about something important?

2. Make a list of your pills, their strength or dosage, and how often you take them, or take them with you. When the doctor asks you what you take, an answer like "One blue pill and three pink ones" isn't helpful.

3. List any herbs or vitamins you take regularly. It is possible that there is an interaction between your regular medications and "natural" things you take that you don't know about. If you don't know why you have been prescribed some medication, now is the time to ask what it is for.

What Your Physical Exam Should Include

The doctor is going to look you over from head to toe. Some feature of your appearance may point immediately to a problem. A hoarse voice, for example, may indicate the need to look further for edema.

During this examination, the doctor will feel all parts of your body, listen to your heart and abdomen with a stethoscope, tap your knees with a tiny rubber hammer to see if you have any neurological problems that could affect your legs, and press your ankles to see if you are retaining fluid. All this will help the doctor assess your overall physical condition.

In addition, this is your opportunity to ask about all those little things that have been bothering you for a while but never enough to call the doctor about. Ask questions about any symptom you have never had before, like pain in your chest or heartburn.

From the Medicine Chest

Be sure you have your yearly vision checkup if ...

◆ You wear contact lenses.

◆ Have a family history of glaucoma.

◆ Have diabetes, hypertension, or take steroids.

◆ Are over 40.

> **CAUTION** **911!**
>
> If you discover something, such as a lump in your breast, or have sudden eye pain or other unexpected symptoms, don't wait. Make an appointment to see your doctor immediately. If you have a high blood pressure reading at the doctor's office, you can monitor it once in a while yourself by using one of those machines you've probably seen in your local drug store. If it continues to be high between doctor visits, give your doctor a call.

From the Medicine Chest

Be sure to keep your yearly skin checkup if …

- You have a family history of skin cancer.
- You have a lot of moles.
- Have a history of frequent burning or tanning.
- Have an already diagnosed skin condition.

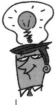

From the Medicine Chest

Be sure to visit your dentist for regular checkups and cleanings, too.

Your physical exam ought to include the following:

- A height and weight exam. If you have gained more than 10 pounds, it is time to do something about it.
- Examination of your thyroid and lymph nodes.
- A hearing screening.
- A vision test.
- An assessment of your heart and neck blood vessels, including blood pressure for a baseline measurement.
- An assessment of your abdomen.
- An assessment of your musculoskeletal system.
- An assessment of your skin.
- An assessment of your neurological system.
- A urinalysis.
- A blood test.

> **CAUTION** **911!**
>
> Hypertension or high blood pressure is called the "silent killer" because it has no symptoms. Fifty million Americans are hypertensive. African Americans are 20 times more likely to be hypertensive than Caucasians. The National Institutes of Health recently changed its view of which number in a blood-pressure reading is the important factor in determining whether a person is hypertensive. Traditionally, diastolic pressure, or the lower number, was thought to be the more important. Now it is the systolic, or higher number in the reading. Blood pressure should be maintained below 140/90 mmHG throughout one's lifetime. A reading higher than this indicates that early therapy is essential.

For Women Only

Your gynecologist may do some of the things your regular doctor does, such as measure your blood pressure and check your weight. In addition, your gynecologist will pay special attention to the following:

- A pelvic exam, including a *pap test*. (After three normal tests, your gynecologist may recommend less frequent exams.)
- A breast exam.
- A urinalysis if there are any indications that you might have an infection or other condition that would warrant one.
- Update of your rubella and tetanus injections.

Every two years:

Women should have a routine checkup with their gynecologist and their regular physician.

At-Risk Women Need Regular or Frequent Pap Tests

If you have had more than one sexual partner or a sexual partner who has had more than one partner; if you have genital warts or an infection with the sexually transmitted human papillomavirus (HPV) disease; are infected with human immunodeficiency virus (HIV); or use tobacco you may need a pap test to detect changes in the cells of the cervix at an early stage.

Ages 45 to 65

Annually:

For women in this age group this checkup should add a cancer screening in addition to all the routine things examined in their regular exam, a urinalysis to check for kidney functioning, and a stool sample to screen for occult

From the Medicine Chest

In the shower while your body is soapy is a good place to examine your breasts for any lumps. You should do this once a month. Make your birthday your routine exam date, that way you won't forget it.

Wellness Words

A **pap test** is a screening test that examines the cells in and around the cervix to detect abnormalities that could lead to cancer. Also called a pap smear, the test is named after Dr. George Papanicolaou, who developed the test in the 1940s.

911!

An estimated 55 percent of U.S. adults are overweight. The National Institutes of Health and statistics from the Behavioral Risk Factor Surveillance System report that obesity constitutes a threefold increased risk for the development of hypertension and diabetes. Watching your weight is about more than looking good.

blood. There is a home occult blood test for blood in the stool now available from your pharmacist or on the Internet. If this test result is positive, your physician can perform a repeat confirming stool sample exam.

Every two years:

◆ A mammogram. (New studies indicate that mammography may not be as effective as once thought, but until something better comes along, women should continue having mammograms.)

Every three years:

◆ A check of blood sugar levels.

◆ A colonoscopy for colon cancer after age 50.

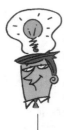

From the Medicine Chest

When you go to the doctor, take along a little notebook and jot down his findings, like your blood pressure reading and how you were told to take your medicine.

Ask for copies of any reports such as bloodwork or urinalysis. If you move or your doctor retires, these records will be very helpful in establishing a new relationship with your new doctor.

Over 65:

Every six months:

◆ A dental exam.

Annually:

This annual exam should now also include a hearing and vision screening with a check for glaucoma.

You might worry if someone in your family has had heart disease or cancer. Doctors are interested in first-degree relatives because these folks share genes with you. If your parents or siblings have had a disease, the likelihood increases that you, too, might be at risk for the disease.

◆ If a lot of your relatives had the same difficulty, heart attacks, or breast cancer, and they came from the same generation, there is a higher chance that you are in jeopardy for the same health problem.

◆ The risk for heart disease and cancer increases with age. Early commencement of these diseases may better reveal the influence of your genetic possibility to be at risk than if your relatives developed the disease late in life.

For Men Only

Age 18 to 39:

♦ A dental exam.

Every two years:

In addition to the regular exam, your checkup should include the following:

♦ A blood count.

♦ An examination of your thyroid, lymph nodes, skin, and testicles.

Every five years:

♦ Add a check for cholesterol.

From the Medicine Chest

You may be feeling great, but it is a good idea to have a regular doctor, a primary-care physician, someone you can call in an emergency or go to when you don't know whether or not to worry about vague symptoms, or someone who will keep you up to date on your immunizations and fill you in on any screening tests you didn't know you might need. If you don't have a regular physician, get one before you need one in an emergency.

Age 40 to 65:

Annually:

For men in this age group, in addition to your regular exam, this checkup should include an examination of the prostate and rectum and may include a *PSA* blood test for prostate cancer. A test for occult blood in the stool should be performed as well, either at home or by your physician.

♦ A dental exam.

♦ A vision check, including test for glaucoma.

Every three years:

♦ A urinalysis to check kidney function.

♦ A check of blood sugar levels.

♦ A colonoscopy after age 50 to screen for colon cancer.

Wellness Words

Prostate specific antigen (PSA) is a blood test that can be helpful in detecting prostate cancer. Although this is a very slow-growing cancer, the American Cancer Society recommends that men over age 50 have a yearly PSA and a rectal examination of the prostate. High-risk groups include those with a family history of the disease and African Americans

Over age 65:

Semi-annually:

- A dental exam.

Annually:

The checkup should now include a stool sample to check for occult blood or a preliminary home test, plus an examination of the rectum.

Every three years:

- A check of blood sugar levels.
- Hearing and vision tests, including a test for glaucoma.

Every 10 years:

- A colonoscopy to screen for colon cancer.

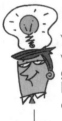

From the Medicine Chest

Your continued good health begins in your mouth. Keep your teeth healthy if you want to keep your health. If you lose your teeth, your ability to chew your food is greatly diminished. People who no longer have their teeth choose food that often lacks nutrients as well as fiber. They may give up all those chewable things like apples and carrots and opt for foods that are easy to swallow without chewing.

For Both Men and Women

- At age 65, an annual flu shot and a one-time pneumonia shot. Most healthy adults only need one pneumonia shot in their lifetime.
- Bring your tetanus shot up to date every 10 years.

In addition to seeing your doctor on a regular basis, you now have access to a number of self-testing medical kits available for purchase at your local pharmacy or on the Internet. These include the following:

- Microcoagulation test for those on long-term anti-coagulation therapy.
- Blood glucose test for Type I and II diabetics who want to check the effectiveness of their diabetic management.

◆ Detection kits for colorectal disorders.

◆ HIV test kits.

If your home-test results are positive, advise your physician.

The Least You Need to Know

◆ A regular physical exam is good preventive medicine to keep small problems from becoming big ones.

◆ Your physical shouldn't be a frightening experience if you go prepared and know what to expect.

◆ A physical exam for women includes a pap test and breast examination.

◆ A physical exam for men includes an examination of the testicles and a test for prostate cancer.

Your Wellness Preparedness Plan

In This Chapter

◆ Wellness preparedness
◆ Your top priorities
◆ When the unexpected happens

Accidents happen, and so do unexpected colds and the flu and even more serious events such as heart attacks and strokes. Illness and injury *always* happen at the most inconvenient times.

Although there are some health matters that are unpreventable, there are many things you can do to help avert disease and maintain wellness. Isn't that a better plan than cure-oriented, crisis-management approach you've been taking so far?

Healthy People 2010, a National Initiative

The Surgeon General challenges individuals, communities, and professionals to take specific steps to ensure that all enjoy good health and long life.

The Surgeon General's Report on Health Promotion and Disease Prevention is a national initiative to improve the health of all Americans through prevention. Its health promotion and disease prevention objectives target a list of 22 areas concerned with being healthy and staying healthy. The office of the Surgeon General has included all of them in a fact sheet aimed at achieving a healthy life for all citizens by the year 2010 as follows:

1. Physical Activity and Fitness
2. Nutrition
3. Tobacco
4. Substance Abuse
5. Family Planning
6. Mental Health
7. Violence
8. Educational and Community-Based Programs
9. Unintentional Injuries
10. Occupational Safety and Health
11. Environmental Health
12. Food and Drug Safety
13. Oral Health
14. Maternal and Infant Health
15. Heart Disease and Stroke
16. Cancer
17. Diabetes and Chronic Disabling Conditions
18. HIV Infection
19. Sexually Transmitted Diseases
20. Immunization and Infectious Diseases
21. Clinical Preventive Services
22. Surveillance and Data Systems

The Surgeon General's list includes physical activity and fitness as the number-one priority for health. Current reports indicate that obesity has become an epidemic and is a recognized prelude to a variety of ailments. Keeping weight within normal limits should be a primary goal for everyone interested in wellness.

Some of the items on the Surgeon General's 22-item list are aimed specifically at community programs rather than individuals, but this list provides an overview of objectives and overall goals that individual wellness preparedness ought to include.

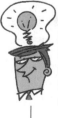

From the Medicine Chest

The Surgeon General provides a four-point prescription that his office would like all of us to follow:

- ◆ Moderate physical activity, at least 5 days a week, 30 minutes a day.
- ◆ Avoid toxins—tobacco, illicit drugs, and abuse of alcohol.
- ◆ Eat at least five servings of fruits and vegetables a day.
- ◆ Responsible sexual behavior and abstinence where appropriate.

Being prepared means having a plan to stay well, to stop little problems from becoming larger ones. It means you also need to prevent or treat an illness or an injury sensibly. It means having the necessary knowledge to know just what you can handle and what you can't and when it is time to call for assistance.

There are health problems that have few or vague warning signs, yet they are some of the major problems that you may have to face while you try to stay healthy.

Know Who You Are

Uncle Charlie or Aunt Liz may or may not be your favorite relatives, but knowing your genetic history has a lot to do with being aware and prepared for the diseases or ailments that might lie waiting in your future. If you have ever filled out one of those questionnaires at the doctor's office that asks whether or not your parents are still living and, if not, what they died from, you are providing clues to the kind of health problems your physician might expect to have concern about for you.

A family history of heart disease, diabetes, hypertension, and cancer indicate that you should be vigilant about your own health goals and concerns. If Uncle Charlie had a heart attack at 45 and your father had one 10 years later, or if Aunt Liz is a diabetic and so is her daughter, you should be aware that these conditions and others tend to run in families, which means you should take extra precautions with your own wellness.

From the Medicine Chest

If anybody knows all the details of your family history, Granny probably does. A visit to see her or a letter might provide you with valuable information about the health and wellness of other relatives, and she will probably be delighted to tell all the family history she knows. Other relatives such as aunts, uncles, or cousins might also be sources of your family's wellness history.

A Heartache Isn't Always Love

Any family history of heart disease should make you aware of the need to be extra vigilant in taking care of your cardiovascular system. Knowing the warning signals of a heart attack, which can cause irreversible injury to the heart muscle, can help keep you safe. Here are the major symptoms of cardiac arrest or a heart attack:

◆ Uncomfortable pressure, fullness, squeezing, or pain in the center of the chest lasting more than a few minutes.

◆ Pain spreading to the shoulders, neck, or arms. The pain may be mild to intense. It may feel like pressure, tightness, burning, or a heavy weight. It may be located in the chest, upper abdomen, neck, jaw, or inside the arms or shoulders.

◆ Chest discomfort with lightheadedness, fainting, sweating, nausea, or shortness of breath. Anxiety, nervousness, and/or cold, sweaty skin. Paleness or pallor.

◆ Increased or irregular heart rate.

◆ A feeling of impending doom.

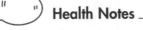

Health Notes

Coronary heart disease is uncommon at total cholesterol levels below 150 milligrams per deciliter. Keep your cholesterol low with diet and exercise as much as possible. Additional cholesterol-lowering medications can be prescribed if your regular test results indicate you need more assistance.

Not all these signs occur in every attack, and sometimes they go away and then come back. Don't wait to see what happens; call 911 right away.

If you have a family history of heart disease, knowledge of heart symptoms, diet, exercise, and a plan of action should be high on your list of priorities in your personal plan to stay well. Others in your workplace and household should know the telephone number and the name of your doctor and what symptoms they should look for if it appears you need emergency help.

More Than a Spoonful of Sugar

A family history of diabetes or weight that is outside of normal limits ought to make you vigilant to being aware of the symptoms that precede this disease. The American Diabetic Association reports that 16 million Americans have diabetes and 5 million don't know it. Diabetes often goes undiagnosed because many of the symptoms seem to be harmless:

◆ Frequent urination

◆ Excessive thirst

◆ Extreme weight loss

- Increased fatigue
- Irritability
- Blurry vision

Any of these symptoms ought to alert you to see your doctor, because early detection will decrease your chance of developing diabetes and its serious complications.

If you are diagnosed with the disease, you should inform yourself about the dietary changes you need to make to stay healthy.

When Steam Doesn't Come Out of Your Ears

Awareness of the potential for high blood pressure to cause major health problems, particularly if you have a family history of the disease or if you are carrying excess weight, should be part of your plan to stay healthy. More than 50 million people in the United States have high blood pressure, including half of women over age 60. High blood pressure or hypertension usually doesn't have any warning signs or symptoms, but it increases your risk for getting heart disease and kidney disease, and for having a stroke.

Most doctors diagnose high blood pressure on the basis of two or more readings taken on different days. A consistent pressure reading of 140/90 mmHG or higher is considered hypertension. You can learn to take your pressure regularly yourself, and most local fire departments will have a paramedic take your pressure—just drop by and ask.

Have your blood pressure checked regularly. If it is high your doctor can prescribe a medication to help keep it under control, explain to you the risks involved in not controlling it, and assist you in developing a plan to lose any excess weight.

> **CAUTION**
>
> **911!**
>
> Don't rely on just one blood pressure reading when it comes to diagnosing high blood pressure. Some people only have high blood pressure when they go to the doctor. It is called *white-coat hypertension*. If your doctor suspects this, you may be asked to wear a device called an ambulatory pressure monitor, which is worn for 24 hours and takes your pressure every 30 minutes.

Take Some Strokes Off Your Game—of Life

The single most important risk factor for stroke is high blood pressure. You may also be more at risk if you are male, African American, have a family history, have been diagnosed with diabetes, sickle cell disease, continue to smoke, and are overweight.

More than 500,000 Americans have a stroke each year, but because of medical advances, the risk of dying is less than half of what it was 20 years ago.

Strokes and transient ischemic attacks (TIAs) often strike without warning. Symptoms may be subtle and painless and may last only a few minutes or seconds, but they are medical emergencies. The most common warning signs are as follows:

- Sudden numbness, weakness, or paralysis of the face, arm, or leg, usually on one side of the body.
- Loss of speech, or trouble talking or understanding speech.
- Dizziness, loss of balance or coordination
- Sudden severe headache
- Difficulty swallowing

Stroke is a serious medical emergency that requires prompt medical attention. Having an awareness of your risk factors; keeping diabetes, high blood pressure, and weight under control; as well as regular use of low-dose aspirin or other blood thinner should be part of your preparedness plan. Have the name and phone number of your physician readily available, and be sure your family members know what to do in an emergency.

Sometimes Think I'm Going Crazy

The National Institute of Mental Health realized that *stressed out*, *anxious*, and *out of control* are words many of us use regularly to describe how we are feeling. Anxiety disorders are the most common mental health problem in the United States. More than 23 million Americans are filled with overwhelming anxiety and fear that is chronic, unremitting, and will grow progressively worse if left untreated.

Sometimes these feelings go on to include subtle changes in every-day, routine life events. Sleepless nights or changes in appetite, for example, may have a variety of differing causes that have little to do with mental health but rather have been affected by external forces that are temporary in nature and probably shouldn't be of concern:

- Loss of a sense of humor
- Sudden feelings of terror that strike without warning
- Repeated, intrusive, and unwanted thoughts
- Nightmares, anger, irritability, and being easily distracted or startled
- Disabling and irrational fear that leads to avoidance of objects or situations
- Exaggerated worry about everyday routine life events and activities

If you find that any of these changes in routine life events last at least six months and are also accompanied by changes in sleep patterns, level of energy, appetite, sex drive, and interpersonal relations, it may be time to seek some help. Talk to your primary physician to see if there are any physical conditions that might be involved in your symptoms and then, if you need more support, get a referral to a mental health professional.

If I Ignore It, It Might Just Go Away

Cancer is a group of diseases that may cause virtually any sign or symptom, but there are some general (nonspecific) signs and symptoms you should be aware of:

♦ Unexplained weight loss of 10 pounds or more, particularly with cancer of pancreas, stomach, esophagus, or lung.

♦ Almost all cancers may produce fever, particularly if it affects the immune system.

♦ Fatigue when the cancer causes a chronic loss of blood as in some colon or stomach cancers.

♦ Pain, particularly in bone or testicular cancer.

In addition to the previous general symptoms, the following are the seven common symptoms that you should always be on the alert for:

♦ A change in bowel habits or bladder function

♦ A sore that does not heal

♦ Unusual bleeding or discharge

♦ Thickening or lump in the breast or other parts of the body

♦ Indigestion or difficulty swallowing

♦ Recent change in a wart or mole

♦ Nagging cough or hoarseness

A family history of any cancer should be cause for you to include an awareness of these symptoms in your wellness preparedness plan. If you experience any one of them, they should be brought to the attention of your doctor right away. Such prompt action may save your life.

But We Love Each Other

Statistics from the Centers for Disease Control's Division of Sexually Transmitted Diseases indicate that one out of every five Americans carries a sexually transmitted disease and four million become infected with chlamydia every year. You are at risk if you have multiple partners or relatively new partners.

A large majority of the sexually transmitted diseases are either without symptoms or the symptoms are mild enough to be ignored until they cause irreversible damage or infertility.

♦ **Chlamydia.** The symptoms are mild or absent.

♦ **Genital herpes.** The symptoms for many people are minimal.

◆ **Genital warts.** There are no early signs.

◆ **Gonorrhea.** Women have no symptoms. Men experience burning on urination.

◆ **Syphilis.** Called the great imitator because the symptoms are indistinguishable from many other diseases.

◆ **Trichomonasis.** Women have a vaginal discharge. Men have no symptoms.

◆ **HIV.** No symptom until seven to nine years after infection.

From the Medicine Chest

Use a new condom for every act of vaginal, anal, and oral sex. Eliminate any air in the tip to keep the condom from breaking. Do not unroll the condom before placing it on the penis. Water-based lubricant on the outside of the condom will reduce the chance of breakage. After removal, wash your hands with soap and water.

Everyone should understand that taking precautions such as using a condom is prudent and sensible. Don't be afraid to discuss your concerns with your sexual partner and exchange information about previous sexual partners for your mutual protection. Don't be embarrassed to ask for STD testing when you get your annual physical. It is sensible to get tested routinely for STDs, because most of us are in denial about whether or not we are at risk until it is too late—and that's the naked truth.

Accidents Happen

According to U.S. Consumer Product Safety Commission statistics, accidents in modern industrial societies happen frequently. Each year in the United States, 1 in 3 people suffers some kind of an injury, and 20 million suffer injury in their own home. Many of these accidents are from common household objects such as garage door openers, bathtubs, toys, toothpicks, pots, pans, hot water, and throw rugs. The list of everyday objects and activities that can and do cause harm is endless. Another 10 million are injured annually in auto related accidents.

It is clear that even the most alert, deliberate, and careful individuals are likely to get hurt occasionally. Since you spend time in the company of co-workers, children, family, and others who are potential sources of accidents and minor emergencies, knowledge of basic first aid is essential for every mature adult.

The American Red Cross suggests that you take an emergency preparedness course so that you feel competent to decide if an injury is serious enough to require medical attention and that you are able to perform CPR and the Heimlich maneuver.

You can learn CPR in one two-hour course. Contact your local fire department to get the details of a training course close to you. Being prepared will mean that you will be competent to assess the event or the injury and make a decision—whether this is a minor event, one that you can take care of yourself, or whether you should call 911 for assistance. Finally, keep a well-stocked and up-to-date first-aid kit in your home.

The Least You Need to Know

- Being prepared is the first step to healthy living.

- Knowing the symptoms of common illnesses prevents little problems from becoming major problems.

- When the unexpected happens, if you are informed and prepared you can take the proper action because you are ready. Being prepared means you can handle unexpected illnesses or injuries because you will already know what you should do.

Chapter 23

Tools to Track Your Progress

In This Chapter

- ◆ Getting it all straight
- ◆ Keeping your food pages
- ◆ Keeping your exercise pages
- ◆ Keeping your stress management pages
- ◆ Putting it all together

Have a goal. Okay, you want to be a rock star, a billionaire, or a dot.com genius. Or maybe you want to look good, feel good, and have plenty of energy and enthusiasm. Either way, you probably can't achieve the first set of goals without the other.

We have all heard that we ought to have goals from our teachers, parents, and coaches, as well as all kinds of other bossy people. As much as you probably agree with these helpful folks, it is easy enough to say, but difficult to do if those goals are vague and not really well defined.

Famous Folks Do It

Oprah Winfrey introduced millions of her viewers of her daytime talk show to the idea of a gratitude journal. Later, lots of these viewers appeared on her show and talked about how much better they feel about their lives since they started keeping their journals. They just began writing down what they like about their lives and what they appreciated about their relationships, their jobs, their families, and their friends. They wrote about what they already have in the way of material possessions, and in so doing, they brought into perspective the good things they have, instead of focusing on the negative.

Creative Folks Do It

In *The Artist's Way* (G.P. Putnam's Sons, 1992), a book read by thousands of creative people and many hoping to be more creative, Julia Cameron asks the reader to write what she calls *morning pages*, *stream-of-consciousness* writing, three longhand pages about whatever comes to mind as soon as you wake up. It is her belief that all the whining you do on those pages, whether it is simple stuff like "I hate doing the laundry," to complaints about your job or family, the very writing about these things helps you start thinking creatively. Cameron believes that these negative thoughts are the thoughts that stand between you and your creative spirit. Writing them down gets them out of the way. After a while, when the morning complaining is all done and you have complained about almost everything, you will begin to write the good stuff.

Real People Do It, Too

Many people have kept personal diaries, some of them since they were small children, recording their innermost thoughts, their hopes, and their dreams in them. Who hasn't practiced writing their some daydreamed-for married name, or their name with "Dr." in front of it?

If you have ever kept a diary or any kind of a journal, then you are already acquainted with the concept of journaling. If you haven't done that, you surely have done some kind of record-keeping, even if it was only doing your (ugh!) tax forms.

A very special part of the brain, the *reticular activating system*, functions as a communication link between the mind and the body. Writing things down makes them concrete in a way that just imagining or thinking about them doesn't. Writing makes it real.

A Four Pillars of Wellness Journal

Your Wellness Journal will be specific to your plan to increase your focus on a healthy lifestyle.

- Purchase a loose-leaf notebook.
- Make copies of the four different pages in this chapter.
- Write a short-term and a long-term goal for each one.
- Take some blank pages with you each day, so you can record things on them as they happen, rather than trying to reconstruct your activities later in the day.

Think It!

Goal-setting is deciding on what you want to accomplish and then moving in small increments toward achieving that goal. Professional athletes often employ a professional psychologist to help them focus on their goals and assist them in visualizing the accomplishment. These athletes are asked to visualize themselves accomplishing their objectives, seeing themselves moving in that direction, and actually doing whatever it takes to become the athlete they want to become.

Write It!

Write down what you think you need to work on. Planning how you are going to accomplish this makes your thinking concrete, not just some wish or dream that some day you will eat properly, jump up in the morning and head for the gym, and by chance or luck you will still be doing that six months or a year from now. Instead, you will have a definite plan that will outline what you need to do every day and a way to look back and see if you have accomplished even a portion of your original plan. If you haven't accomplished what you planned, it is time to reevaluate. Did you make it too difficult? Too easy? You can look back and see what you need to revise and continue setting new goals.

Do It!

Nobody likes to write an outline because it seems much easier to just plunge into the job and try to get it done. Sometimes, at the end of all that work, you may discover that an outline (if you're a writer), a cost plan (if you're an architect), or a recipe (if you're a cook) would have kept you on track. A plan will show you before you get started that the plot, the building materials, or the ingredients aren't all there. Focusing only on an outcome without proper ingredients lined up is a recipe for failure. A goal with a plan will highlight the weaknesses and strengths in your wellness project, the creation of a well you, before you start.

Success will make you able to move on to the next step in your goals. By focusing on short- and then long-term goals you will be able to develop a definite plan. Such a plan will decrease your anxiety and improve your confidence that you can achieve wellness.

Health Notes

In 1992, decathlon athlete Dan O'Brien couldn't stop negative thinking and didn't qualify for the U.S. Olympic team. With the help of a sports psychologist he refocused, replacing negative thoughts with reassuring ones, and won that long-hoped for Olympic gold.

Accentuate the Positive

Write a brief outline of your plan, including your goals, listing what you plan to accomplish. As you work through this outline, reward yourself with some words of praise as a small token of your appreciation of your efforts, something that will remind you every time you think about it or see it of a step well done.

◆ Decide if you are going to begin with a four-week plan or a three-month one. While it is easier to write the same plan for three months, you will be more precise in the details, able to see how much you have accomplished sooner, and will get satisfaction earlier from completing a shorter plan.

◆ Begin by writing your goals as a positive statement. It is better to write "I will begin each week by creating my healthy shopping list" rather than "I will try and leave potato chips off my shopping list." Or "I'm going to designate a particular place where I will always put my glasses, my keys, and my umbrella" rather than "I need to do something about how forgetful I'm getting."

◆ When you see that you have accomplished one of your goals, enjoy it. Tell yourself how proud you are of you.

◆ Reward yourself with a small token of appreciation for your accomplishment, for example, a new scarf, a movie, or a phone call to an old friend.

Let's Go Shopping

You already know that it isn't a good idea to shop for food when you're hungry. A menu for the next week's meals will help you discover what you need to buy. Sit down and write out a week's food shopping list before you head for the grocery store. If you are familiar with the layout of the grocery store where you regularly shop, you know where the cookies and candy are, so write your list so you don't have to go down those aisles.

A week's shopping list will also help you avoid that last-minute rush to pick up something you forgot. We all know what happens then: You're hungry, you're in a hurry, and that table near the store's checkout stacked with packaged doughnuts looks tempting—a quick snack happens.

It is no accident that bread and milk are kept at the very back of grocery stores. Merchandisers know that if you have to travel through the store to get these items, you probably will pick up something else you see on your way. If you must pick up some of these staples between your major shopping trips, write them down, even if it is only two items. This will help you focus before you go in to the store to avoid impulse buys.

Four Pillars of Wellness: Food

One-Month Goal Statement

_____

_____

_____

_____

One-Week Goal Statement

_____

Day of the Week	Foods Planned	Foods Eaten	Water
_____	_____	_____	_____
_____	_____	_____	_____
_____	_____	_____	_____
_____	_____	_____	_____
_____	_____	_____	_____
_____	_____	_____	_____
_____	_____	_____	_____
_____	_____	_____	_____

End of week evaluation notes: _____

_____

New goal: _____

Review the chart for the week and see if there are problem areas and focus on positive ways to change them. If you had a snack that you really didn't want but you just ate it because you were bored, write out some of the things you could do the next time before you made a decision to eat that snack. Example: Buy a book of crossword puzzles and put it on the kitchen counter. Next time you're tempted to eat, do a puzzle instead.

From the Medicine Chest

Visualize yourself succeeding. See yourself eating a carrot instead of a cookie. If you learned anything from the first week of keeping food pages, write it down in a proactive form. This will help shape your thoughts, making them much more powerful in your life while giving you positive reinforcement.

A Foodaholic's Tale

Margo, the mother of five, all under the age of 12, is a good cook, and she prides herself on putting decent meals on the table.

"My kids are good eaters," she says with pride. "They will try new things and they usually eat all their vegetables. My problem is snacks. They come running in after school looking for something to eat. They want cookies or brownies or even one of those small boxes of cereal. These occasional snacks for active children are one thing, but the problem for me began when I started to eat some of them myself, just because they were there." Margo laughed, "I have finally figured out what to do. I bring cookies home, or I bake them myself. I close them in Baggies, put them inside an *opaque* container and put that container on the top shelf of the pantry. Remember that old saying, 'out of sight, out of mind?' Well, it works. I don't think about them because I don't see them. If I decide I want one, I have to climb up there, open that container, open the Baggie and then put it all back. It isn't worth it. Before I get half way there, I opt for fresh cut veggies that I already have in the refrigerator."

Let's Exercise

If you have ever joined a gym, you have seen the little cards they make out that help you keep track of your progress. Most of these cards divide your workouts into two sections: cardiovascular and strength. Even if you have no intention of joining a gym but plan to bike, swim, play soccer with friends, or tennis at the club, it will be helpful if you will keep a record of what you are doing and also to take a look at whether your chosen sport is neglecting some part of your physical self.

For example, bike riding, is a lot of fun and terrific exercise, but it does very little for your upper body. You need to plan to do something else to take care of your arms, chest, and shoulders.

Harry, a long-haul trucker says, "I just sort of fell into getting soft and pudgy. After a minor accident to my knee, I sat around, drinking a few beers, surfing the TV channels, and watching other guys play sports. I used that knee injury as an excuse. After it was better, I continued to use it to be lazy.

"One of my buddies was getting married and asked me to be the best man. When I saw their wedding album I was absolutely horrified to see this huge balloon of a guy standing next to the groom. I couldn't believe that person was me. Although I look in the mirror on a regular basis, it took a photo with normal-size people to make me wake up, to realize I had to do something *NOW*.

Four Pillars of Wellness: Exercise

One-Month Goal Statement

_____

_____

_____

_____

One-Week Goal Statement

_____

Day of the Week	Exercise Cardio Strength	Plan	Duration Actual
_____	_____	_____	_____
_____	_____	_____	_____
_____	_____	_____	_____
_____	_____	_____	_____
_____	_____	_____	_____
_____	_____	_____	_____
_____	_____	_____	_____
_____	_____	_____	_____

End of week evaluation notes: _____

_____

New goal: _____

_____

"I put pictures from that wedding in the front of my Wellness Journal. I sat down and wrote out my goals and got started. It took a few weeks, but my body began to change. I could see it, and people I work with saw it, too. Everybody began asking me what I was doing." Harry smiled, "They all laughed at me and everybody said, 'Yeah, I've started on exercise programs a couple of hundred times myself and you know what happened? Nothing. After a few weeks I went back to being the old slob I was before. You'll probably do the same, Harry.'

"I understood what they were saying. The difference for me is that this time I wrote out some goals and made a plan about what I was going to do and how I was going to do it."

From the Medicine Chest

Locate some recent photos of yourself taken at a party or at the beach. They don't have to be of you in a bathing suit. In fact, if you look in that old shoe box on the top shelf of your closet for photos you will probably find you kept the ones where you think you look pretty good. Looking good, looking fat, looking terrible, looking sickly—it really doesn't matter, but you can use any recent photo to keep you in touch with the person you were when you began your wellness journey. Stick those photos in your journal so you will have something to remind you about who you were as you go on your journey to being a person who has decided on *wellness* as a way of life.

Yikes! It Drives Me Crazy!

Everyone has their own definition of stress. There are people who say they actually like stress and call stress challenging.

If you have never thought about what stress means to you, a few weeks of keeping a Wellness Journal will help you define it for yourself. Most of us dislike arguments and will go out of our way to avoid confrontations, but there are people for whom that kind of a life is actually fun. You know them; they eventually go on to become lawyers.

There are all kinds of occupations where extreme stress is often part of the daily workplace: fire fighters, police officers, and critical care nurses, to name a few. There are people others might consider risk-takers, skiers who whoosh down a run at 70 miles per hour, those who think sky diving is entertaining, and others who wrestle alligators or milk venomous snakes. For the majority of us, however, just living in today's world with high-pressure work environments, money worries, problems with relationships or lack of relationships can be stressful, and the urge to fight or run has to be suppressed.

As a part of the fight-or-flight response to anything you see as a stressor, your stress hormones immediately respond. They rev up your heart and blood vessels, your immune system, your lungs, your digestive system, your sensory organs, and your brain. Your hormones get all your systems ready to go. Unless you know what your stressors are and take some action to reduce or deal with them, they will drive you crazy and eventually make you physically ill.

Four Pillars of Wellness: Stress

One-Month Goal Statement

_____

_____

_____

_____

One-Week Goal Statement

_____

Record your stress hourly and give the stress you are feeling a rating on a scale from 1 to 10. Briefly record what happened, where (work/driving/home), what your response was (yelled/laughed/walked away), then the new action you are going to take the next time a similar situation arises (listen/talk quietly/agree to help).

Day/Time	Stressor Event	Scale (1 to 10)	Response	Action Taken
_____	_____	_____	_____	_____
_____	_____	_____	_____	_____
_____	_____	_____	_____	_____
_____	_____	_____	_____	_____
_____	_____	_____	_____	_____
_____	_____	_____	_____	_____
_____	_____	_____	_____	_____
_____	_____	_____	_____	_____

End of week evaluation notes: _____

_____

New goal: _____

_____

A Grump's Tale

Barney, a self-described computer geek, didn't think he had a problem. "I am the kind of guy who prides himself on being able to roll with the punches, and there have been a few of them in my life that haven't been easy to take." Barney shrugged, "I guess everyone has their ups and downs, and I'm no different. It was a road-rage incident that made me realize I was getting out of control. I was so mad that I chased this guy off the interstate and had every intention of forcing him off the road and punching his lights out. I was trembling all over, sweating, and swearing. When I finally caught up to the car, the driver turned out to be a very tiny old lady. She gave me a sweet smile as I pulled up along side her. It was obvious she didn't have a clue."

"I realized in that moment that I had lost my sense of humor and lost my patience with other people, including my boss, my wife, my children, and my in-laws.

"I went to see my doctor because I thought I was going to have a heart attack. He told me that I better get control of myself or that was exactly what was going to happen. That was easy for him to say, but not so easy for me to figure out. I absolutely *had* to find a new way to look at events in my life.

"Keeping the Stress Journal has made it possible for me to see what gets me fired up, how I have handled it in the past, and what changes I must make to handle things differently.

"I'm working on the sense of humor thing right now. Mine is a high-pressure computer job, and I have learned that if I react with frustration it only gets worse. That has been my *response* style. Now I need a new *action* style. I stop, take a couple of deep breaths, and try to see if I can find something funny in the situation. Sometimes that isn't so easy, but other times within a few minutes I can see how ridiculous it all is and I can laugh. I feel a lot better right away."

Four Pillars of Wellness: Prevention

It may take you a little while to see a pattern, but you will find that sometimes your stress response has been to eat when you weren't hungry or cancel your workout so you can sulk or brood over a minor incident or thoughtless remark from someone at work. If you got frustrated waiting in line while some idiot counted out her change, and your stress level went up over that, it will show up in your journal pages.

Take your current food, exercise, and stress journal pages and lay them out side-by-side. You can now record items in the two separate parts for your prevention pages.

1. Record the connection you discover between your stress and your food consumption, your food consumption and your stress, your exercise or lack of it and stress and food. What steps you plan to short-circuit this cycle then becomes a part of your prevention plan.

2. Write a brief paragraph about your response to the connections you found and your plan to avoid this connection triggering the same response again.

Once you have identified the sources of your stress and changes in your food or exercise goals and begin to change your usual responses from negative to proactive, you are on the road to finding methods for managing your health and staying well. When you have identified the events that create a situation that trigger anger or anxiety, or a negative physical response such as a headache or an upset stomach, you can begin to change those situations, and as a result, you will find that your eating habits will improve, your exercise regime can then contribute to relaxation, and all your wellness techniques and steps toward that goal will become easier to follow.

Because your eating patterns, exercise routines, and stressors are unique to you and you alone and they are intertwined, a well-kept Pillars of Wellness Journal is going to be your personalized roadmap to health. It will work like no other that you have read about in any book, seen on television, or heard about from a friend. It may take a little more work, but it will be one that you have prepared and created for yourself.

Four Pillars of Wellness

One-Month Goal Statement

_____
_____
_____
_____

One-Week Goal Statement

Food/Exercise	Date	Stress Connection	Prevention Plan
_____	_____	_____	_____
_____	_____	_____	_____
_____	_____	_____	_____
_____	_____	_____	_____
_____	_____	_____	_____
_____	_____	_____	_____
_____	_____	_____	_____
_____	_____	_____	_____

Wellness paragraph for week of: _____

Wellness paragraph for the month of: _____
_____

The Least You Need to Know

- Keeping a Wellness Journal will define targets and goals.
- Keeping food pages will help you focus on what you eat, when you eat, and snacking habits that need adjustment to aid you in making changes in your eating habits.
- Keeping exercise pages will help you see how much time you spend exercising, the kind of exercise you do, and will help you plan your time.

◆ Keeping stress pages will help you know what stresses you, how you can plan to defuse those stressors, and find new ways to keep your stress level down.

◆ Putting it all together makes it possible for you to get an overview of your four pillars of wellness and what you can do to make it all come together into a cohesive plan that is uniquely yours.

Part 6

Wrapping It Up

Well, you've done it. You've learned just about everything about wellness that we could cram into these pages. Now the question is ... what are you going to do about it?

We've all got great intentions. There's hardly one of us who hasn't rushed out to buy the latest fitness video or fad diet book or who hasn't invested good money to buy a treadmill or stair-stepper that ends up serving more as a fancy clothes hanger than a fitness tool.

Reading about wellness is one thing; incorporating that knowledge into the fabric of our everyday lives is quite another. In this part, we'll give you some tools to help you make the behaviors that promote and support wellness as natural to you as breathing.

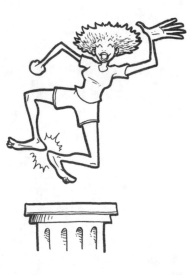

Chapter 24

You Deserve It—Convincing Yourself That Wellness Is Important

In This Chapter

- ◆ Who's number one?
- ◆ Taking care of yourself
- ◆ The importance of scheduling
- ◆ The differences between success and failure

Now that you've taken in all this knowledge about wellness, what are your plans? Do you intend to start a program incorporating the things you have learned to enhance your own wellness? Or are you going to sit back on your haunches, shrug, say, "That's nice," put the book down, and then go on about your merry, wellness-destroying way?

It's a big, important question, and you are the only one who can answer it for yourself. Before you decide, let's look at where you stand in your own scheme of things. Maybe then we can give you a few pointers to boost your estimation of your own importance.

Do You Put Yourself First or Last?

In our modern world, self-sacrifice seems to be a buzzword, particularly for mothers. Self-sacrifice is well and good, but not if you're sacrificing your own needs to the extent that you're endangering your health.

If you are last on your own list, you can hardly expect anyone else to step up and help you or treat you better than you treat yourself. Embarking on a wellness program is all about setting priorities. If you don't think you're important enough to deserve the best possible care, then no one else will think so, either. If you treat yourself with courtesy, respect, and consideration, then others will treat you the same way. If you ignore the needs of your body and mind for care, comfort, and renewal, you are setting yourself up for illness in the not too distant future. It's that simple.

There was a famous case in Houston, Texas, a few years ago where a mother nursed her husband and each of her six children through a virulent, life-threatening strain of the flu. She knew she was sick, too, but took no treatment, didn't go see a doctor herself, or even mention her symptoms to her children's doctor when she took them in. Ill though she was, she sacrificed sleep, food, and medicine, all in the name of taking care of her family. When the last one of them was well, she finally took herself to the doctor, barely able to breathe and feeling worse than she had ever felt in her life. While sitting in that crowded waiting room, the young mother keeled over dead. It made the front page of all the local newspapers. She had been straining so hard to draw a breath that she ruptured a blood vessel in her lungs and bled to death before anyone could help her.

In her quest to care for her family, this mother ignored her own needs and ended up abandoning the very people she loved most in the whole world. If only she had loved herself a little better!

Don't let yourself end up in a bad situation simply because you fail to take action to protect your own health and well-being. Putting yourself first is not a sin; it's a necessity if you want to achieve true wellness.

Self-Sacrifice Can Be Self-Defeating

We tell you this tragic story for a reason. There's a time when self-sacrifice becomes self-defeating. If you are ignoring your own needs in favor of caring for your family, you're not doing anyone any favors. How can you keep caring for the ones you love if you're no longer here?

Although this example may strike you as extreme, anyone who consistently ignores their own health needs because they feel as if the needs of their family are more important should seriously rethink their priorities. Why do you think airlines tell parents to put on their oxygen masks first in case of an emergency? It's because adults are more capable of handling frightening situations and making difficult decisions than children. If all the adults on a plane put masks on their children first, by the time the plane made an emergency landing, there would be no one to open the escape hatches because all the adults would have passed out from oxygen deprivation.

See? Self-defeating.

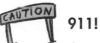

911!

If you're having a medical problem, seek treatment right away. Many people end up with serious health threats because they wait, thinking a problem will go away. For example, don't ignore the first warning signs of cancer. By waiting to seek treatment, you might let your cancer grow from Stage 1 to Stage 3, from curable to life-threatening. If your diagnosis is bad news, at least you will have given yourself the best possible chance by seeking early treatment.

Enlightened Self-Preservation

What you need to do is to enforce a policy of enlightened self-preservation, where you consistently put yourself first. It's not because you're greedy or uncaring, but because you know you're best qualified to care for your family and you love them enough to want to make sure you'll be around to care for them for a long time. If you don't make yourself number one, nobody else is going to. Nobody else can make sure you eat right, get enough sleep, exercise regularly, drink enough water, and take good care of yourself. That's your job. In fact, it's the most important job you will ever have, and you shouldn't neglect it.

The next time you're tempted to make a foolish self-sacrifice in the name of love, look in the mirror and remind yourself, "I'm number one!" Think of a compromise that serves both your needs and the needs of the person you are caring for, and stop automatically putting yourself last. This isn't *Wild Kingdom*, where the lioness makes the kill and then steps back and doesn't eat until after the lion has had his fill. This is modern-day America. You deserve the best life has to offer, and you're the only one who can make sure you get it. And you're the only one who can make yourself believe you're worth it.

The Care and Feeding of ... You

Now that you've realized you're number one, how are you going to take care of this very important person? First, you have to decide that wellness is an important and desirable life goal.

Do You Really Want to Be Well?

Here's a little quiz to help you determine if wellness is something you truly want or not. Circle your preferred answer.

Would you rather have:

1. a. A strong, healthy body

   b. A weak and feeble body

2. a. A slender, trim body

   b. A flabby body

3. a. Lots of energy

   b. Little or no energy

4. a. Excellent health, rarely sick

   b. Poor health, always sick

5. a. An upbeat, positive outlook on life

   b. A downbeat, defeated, depressed outlook

This one is easy to score. If you have all or mostly A's, then you would like to live the wellness lifestyle. If you have all B's, well, gee, why did you buy this book? We think it's because, deep down, you really do want to embrace the good, healthy life.

If, as we suspect, you would like to take good care of yourself, you've taken the first step by buying and reading this book. Now sit down and make a game plan for incorporating wellness into the rest of your life.

Setting Goals

Don't try to change everything all at once. If you're pretty good about exercising but know your diet could use some work, start with improving your nutrition. If you eat right but battle stress constantly and never find the time to exercise, work on exercise first, because exercise helps to relieve stress. Then, when you have regular exercise worked into your routine, try some of the stress management techniques outlined in Part 5, "The Fourth Pillar—Preventive Maintenance," if stress is still a problem for you.

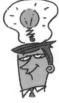

From the Medicine Chest _____

If you don't write down your goals and desired outcomes, you'll greatly reduce your chances of success. An unwritten goal falls more into the category of wishful thinking than a true objective. Writing down goals forces you to visualize the steps that would be necessary to achieve that goal. Visualizing how to achieve a goal is the first step toward realizing success. So be sure to write down your goals and be as specific as possible about what you want to do and the time frame in which you'd like to accomplish it.

Write down the behaviors you would like to incorporate into your life. Post them on your bathroom mirror, refrigerator door, or the wall of your office—wherever you'll be sure to see them daily. When you have successfully adopted a new behavior (meaning that you've passed the 21-day mark and it has become a new and good habit), plan some sort of small celebration.

For example, if you used several stress reduction techniques to get a handle on your daily stress, you might buy yourself a new relaxation CD or a small fountain for your desktop. Maybe you want to indulge in some luxurious bath products or a weekend day trip to that landmark right up the road that you've never had time to visit.

The point is to make the celebration fit the achievement. Make it something that is meaningful to you, something that will encourage you to continue in your quest for the wellness lifestyle.

As you reach your objectives, be sure to add new goals to your list so that your forward progress doesn't stall out. For example, if your goal is to be able to walk one mile comfortably, once you reach that goal you should next try to walk a mile and a half comfortably and so on until you reach the three-mile mark. Once you hit three miles, you might want to up the intensity a bit. Instead of walking at 3 miles per hour, try walking at 3.5 miles per hour. You can use a pedometer or stopwatch to help you measure your speed. Or alternate walking with short bursts of light jogging to get your heart rate into your target zone.

Sticking to It

There will come a day when you have reached all your wellness goals and are just coasting. You've lost the weight and inches you wanted to lose, lowered your blood pressure and bad cholesterol levels, and learned how to let stress roll off you like water off a duck's back. So now what?

Now is the most critical time of all. Now is the time to remind yourself that you have to stick with your wellness-enhancing behaviors to maintain all the gains you've achieved.

Health Notes

Norman Vincent Peale, considered to be the Father of Positive Thinking, once said: "People become really quite remarkable when they start thinking they can do things. When they believe in themselves, they have the first secret of success."

A day or two off the wagon won't hurt. But if you suddenly realize that a big deadline has kept you out of the gym for two weeks and your middle is looking a little like tapioca pudding, you've got to get yourself back on track or risk losing all the gains you've made.

Don't castigate. Don't recriminate. You're human and you got a little sloppy. It won't help for you to shred yourself mercilessly. Falling off the wellness wagon is only a big deal if you let the sloppiness overtake and eliminate the new wellness behaviors you've been practicing.

Do whatever you have to do to motivate yourself, but get your health-enhancing behaviors back in place as quickly as possible. Remember, you're number one, and you deserve to have the best that life has to offer. So get going!

Make a Date with Yourself

Okay, you've read all the books and watched all the videos, but you're still not exercising or eating right. What's the problem? The problem might be that you've forgotten to schedule wellness behaviors into your day.

Get out your planner or calendar or Palm Pilot and take a realistic look at your upcoming week. If you want to spend an hour at the gym three days this week, write it down just as if it was an important business appointment, because guess what? It *is* an important appointment—about the business of keeping yourself fit and well.

If you want to meditate for 20 minutes a day, how could you hope to squeeze that activity in unless you planned for the time in advance?

If you want to eat healthy, green salads for lunch but all the restaurant in your office building serves at lunch is greasy burgers and fries, you're going to have to do some scheduling to stick to your eating plan.

First, decide how long it will take you to assemble and pack the ingredients for a delicious homemade salad. Next, look at your schedule to see where you might realistically fit in that time. Let's say you have determined it would take you 15 minutes to wash and dry your greens, slice your vegetables, mix your salad dressing, then package everything for lunch. If you're a morning person, schedule the time before you leave for work. Get up 15 minutes early or juggle other priorities to fit it in. If you're a night person, schedule the time for right before you go to bed.

Once you get the hang of this sort of scheduling, you'll find additional ways to save time. For example, if you follow the advice in Chapter 9, "Planning Healthy Snacks and Meals," you'll find that you can wash, dry, and package your greens, slice and package your vegetables, and mix your salad dressing for the entire week all in the course of 30 or 40 minutes on a Sunday afternoon or evening. Then all you would have to schedule into your workday is the two or three minutes it takes to walk to the refrigerator before you leave for work and grab the salad package for that day's lunch.

Planning for Everything

Everything you want to do in the course of a day should be scheduled in your planner. How do you honestly hope to find an hour to get to the gym in the middle of a busy day unless you plan in advance to set aside the required time?

You won't, which means you won't get to the gym, and then you'll feel like a failure, and to make yourself feel better, you'll stop and get a triple fudge sundae. See how problems escalate when you don't plan ahead?

By writing down your important wellness activities in your planner, you tell yourself that you're serious about this wellness business. You have goals, and you have a plan, and you aren't going to let anything distract you from reaching those goals.

If you're having trouble with this idea, ask yourself how an important client or business associate would react if you scheduled an appointment with them and then just didn't bother to show up. You should treat your wellness appointments with yourself with the same serious regard. Don't schedule it unless you mean to keep it.

Success or Failure: It's All in Your Mind

When researchers look at people who have succeeded in sticking to improvement programs and compare them to those who have failed, they always find the same important differences in the two groups.

People who are successful usually say they have had some sort of epiphany just before embarking on the successful program. For example, a woman who had 80 pounds to lose had tried and failed at many diets and exercise programs. She was miserably unhappy in her body and couldn't think of anything short of surgery she hadn't tried to lose weight. Except for one thing—self-discipline. As she approached her thirtieth birthday and realized she was getting ready to blow out of misses sizes into the plus-size department, something inside her head just snapped. She knew she didn't want to be an old fat person, and she knew that losing weight only became more difficult as you aged and your metabolism slowed down.

Health Notes

John F. Kennedy said, "There are risks and costs to a program of action. But they are far less than the long range risks and costs of comfortable inactions."

From that day on, she was a woman possessed. Whereas before she would always find an excuse to put the doughnut in her mouth, now she passed. In the past, there wasn't any inducement that could make her exercise, now there wasn't anything that could get her off the treadmill. She did three exercise videos a day when she first started because she wanted to see fast results. It didn't matter to her that at the beginning she could only get through 10 or 15 minutes of an hour-long workout before she collapsed in a chair, gasping for breath. She wasn't judging her results at that point, only her effort. As long as she did her best and didn't give up, she was happy.

Once this woman lost a significant amount of weight, she added strength training to her routine. At the end of 14 months, she had gone from a size 18 to a size 4, and all that had changed was that she put herself and her body's needs first. She scheduled fitness into her day and didn't let anybody blow her off track. Finally, she didn't diet, but she simply substituted healthful food for junk food and started cooking that way for her whole family.

Today, she eats just about anything she wants but watches her portion size and has completely eliminated all junk and fast food from her nutritional plan. She exercises for an hour five days a week, doing a half-hour of cardiovascular work and a half-hour of weight training. She went from fitness failure to success because she discovered her health and happiness were worth the effort. Once she put her wellness needs first in her own mind and wrote down her goals and a time frame to accomplish those goals, the self-discipline to achieve those goals came to her naturally.

Are you ready to discover the source of your own inspiration? Read on and we'll help you figure out what sort of motivation works best for you.

The Least You Need to Know

♦ If you don't make yourself number one, nobody else will.

♦ When you set your priorities, allow enough time for taking good care of your own wellness needs.

♦ If you want to successfully incorporate wellness behaviors into your life, you have to schedule them into your daily routine.

♦ Writing goals down can mean the difference between success and failure.

25

Motivation—a Matter of Carrots and Sticks

In This Chapter

- ◆ What gets you going?
- ◆ Positive or negative motivation
- ◆ The power of visualization
- ◆ Overcoming negative thinking
- ◆ Do you need a wellness partner?

Motivation is a matter of individual preference and personality; what makes you get up and get going may be the very thing that knocks someone else off-course. It's also important to distinguish between real motivation and day-dreaming. In this chapter, we'll help you determine whether you're motivated more by reward or punishment and show you how to master the fine art of self-motivation.

What Motivates You?

Before you start your wellness program, you should try to determine what sort of *motivation* you respond to. Some of us do better when we know there's a reward or a "carrot" waiting at the end of a task. Others do their best not for hope of a reward but in order to avoid a negative consequence or "stick."

Whether we are aware of it or not, almost all of our conscious behavior is motivated by either a positive desire to obtain something we think is beneficial or a negative desire to avoid something we think is detrimental. We have certain needs and desires, both positive and negative, and thinking about those needs leads to planning, which leads to taking whatever actions we think might help us achieve our goals or avoid unpleasant consequences.

Wellness Words

Motivation is what gets you to perform an action. It is the bridge between an idea and its fruition. Motivation makes you put ideas into action. If you have motivation, you act because you want to, not because you have to.

There have been numerous books written on positive versus negative motivation. Researchers have spent hundreds of thousands of dollars of government grant money trying to figure out what makes people tick, only to figure out what most of us already knew or at least suspected—that variations in our motivation produce big differences in our performance. In other words, if we are truly committed to a goal, our likelihood of success will be greater than if we just feel sort of "so-so" about the whole thing.

Are You Really Motivated?

If differences in motivation create such huge differences in results, then what creates those differences in motivation? A lot of it has to do with how we approach our desired goal. If we just lie around and say, "Yeah, I'd like to be fit one day," our chances of actually becoming fit are very small, because we haven't fantasized about any of the steps required to make our dream become a reality. We're not really committed to making any changes in our oh-so-comfortable lifestyles; we're just doing some wishful thinking.

On the other hand, if we are truly motivated, that motivation will translate into commitment, and that commitment will translate into a sort of "mission statement" we can use to define the path to our goals. For example: "This is January, and I'd like to be fit by the time of my high school reunion in July. That means I have to lose 25 pounds, which means I need to rethink my nutrition and start exercising regularly."

Defining a desired goal in this fashion, breaking it down into the steps required to make it become a reality, and making a game plan to perform those steps means you have a much higher chance of being successful in reaching that goal.

Remember, you cannot think your way to success simply by indulging in wishful thinking, but you can think your way to success by setting a goal and then outlining all the steps you must take in order to reach that goal.

From the Medicine Chest _____

One of the simplest ways to remind yourself of your goal is by writing it down in a mission statement that defines exactly what it is you want to accomplish within a particular time frame. Once you are satisfied with your statement, make several copies and tape it up in the places where you are most likely to see it several times a day— on your refrigerator, bathroom mirror, by your treadmill, or by stationary bike. Reading your mission statement several times each day will help to keep you focused on your goal and enhance your chances of success.

The Triggering Event

Ever read about someone who went on diet after diet, tried every exercise plan and every pill, and still didn't meet their weight management goals? Or perhaps you know someone who was determined to organize their office, so they went out and bought books and videos, put up cue cards, shoved a few boxes and stacks of paper around, got frustrated, and then quit. All the books they bought on organization only ended up adding to their clutter.

Take any subject, any goal you can imagine, and we bet you'll be able to think of at least one or two family members or friends who have tried to meet that goal and failed. When you talk to people who have experienced this, you almost always discover that they didn't actually stick to any of their game plans for very long. They half-heartedly tried this and then that but never truly stuck to one plan long enough to give it a chance to work.

Why? Because they were not yet truly motivated to succeed. They were more than happy to talk about their goals, sometimes in grandiose terms, but they couldn't be bothered to make a plan and take the steps necessary to make their goal become reality.

That is, until they experience some sort of triggering event. Someone makes an unkind remark, they have an accident or embarrassing incident related to their size, they get sick due to poor diet or chronic stress, or they miss the filing deadline on a large insurance reimbursement because the necessary paperwork is buried somewhere on their desks. Whatever the cause, people who have succeeded at weight loss, money management, organization, or just about anything will tell you they went from chasing failure to chasing success when they had just such an epiphany. They call it their "life-defining moment," the moment when they decided they had finally had enough of failure and were ready to succeed. You see these types of stories all the time in fitness magazines, and the theme of a life-changing epiphany or triggering event runs through all of them.

◆ "I had to buy two airline seats because I couldn't fit into one, and I finally had enough. I decided something had to change."

You see the same thing in business magazine interviews with people who have enjoyed phenomenal success in one venture or another. It's not unusual to read that these people tried and failed at business after business, never feeling truly passionate, never really giving their all to the cause. Then all of a sudden, something snapped and their hearts and minds changed. They found something they really liked to do, they made a great plan, they followed the plan to the letter, and—surprise, surprise!—the success that had eluded them for so long was suddenly theirs.

◆ "I tried multi-level marketing, a fast-food franchise, and even went into business with my brother, but nothing worked. I finally had enough and decided something had to change."

"I finally had enough." These are words not of defeat but of determination, words of decision. They are your way of saying to the world (and to yourself) that you know whatever it is that you've been doing isn't working, and you know you've got to make some real changes if you ever want to see real results.

Have you finally had enough? If so, you're ready to make the changes that will make wellness an integral part of your daily life. If not, we have a few ideas to help you figure out your motivational style. Once you understand that, you'll know just what sort of fire you need to light under yourself to get going.

Find Your Motivational Style

One thing we know for sure is that life is never static. We always seem to be spiraling up, building step-by-step toward some goal, or spiraling down, sliding inch-by-inch toward failure. We don't stay in the same place for long.

In order to understand how to motivate yourself, you must first determine whether you are more influenced by positive outcomes, or carrots, or by the fear of negative outcomes, or sticks, whether you see the cup as half-full or half-empty.

Health Notes

Henry Ford is famous for many things, but not this quote. Nonetheless, it's worth repeating here. "Whether you think that you can or that you can't, you are usually right." In other words, you create your own destiny with the power of your thoughts.

The Half-Full Cup

People who are motivated by positive outcomes do not unduly fear the consequences of potential failure. They are optimists by nature and believe they can accomplish almost anything they want. Once they have set their mind on achieving a goal, they will do their level best to attain that objective. They concentrate their thinking on the benefits of reaching their goal: fitting back into a size 10, getting compliments from people who notice their trim, new shape, feeling better, and having more energy. They don't waste much time asking themselves "But what if ...?" They work for recognition, advancement, prestige, a sense of achievement, and pride in a job well done. If they fail, they get right back up again and start anew.

The problem with optimists is that they have trouble trying to get settled on one objective. They like to flit from one idea and project to another, drawing a lot of energy and satisfaction simply from talking about a projected goal. They have to move from the "talking about it" to the "doing it" stage, and that can be their biggest tripping point.

Optimists require a gentle hand to stay motivated and on target. Just let someone yell at them or present them with a long list of onerous rules they must stick to "or else," and they will fold their tents and run away.

The Half-Empty Cup

People who are motivated by negative outcomes do not think about the good that might come if they are successful in meeting their goals. They worry about the bad that might come if they are not. They are afraid they might have a heart attack or stroke, so they get on the treadmill and walk for an hour every day, not because they enjoy exercise or joyfully anticipate what life will be like when they are fit and trim. They exercise because they are terrified of what might happen to them if they keep sitting in their recliners.

If you're motivated by fear of negative outcomes and happen to engage a fitness trainer who is Little Miss Sunshine, who bounces all over the place, clapping her hands in glee and telling you how *grr-r-r-eat* life is going to be once you reach your training goal, her message will fall on deaf ears. In fact, after a few sessions, you may feel like bench-pressing Little Miss Sunshine.

If however, you get General Patton as your trainer, a guy who yells at you and swears you will keel over dead if you miss so much as one day of exercise, you've found your match, a person whose style will motivate you to achieve your goals.

If fear is what motivates you, there is no sense lamenting your fate. Use that self-knowledge to help you reach your goals.

We Can't All Be Alike

It's counterproductive to insist that everyone adapt the same motivational style; one is not necessarily better than the other. What is important is to figure out what your own style is, because that will help you motivate yourself.

Here's a short quiz to help you determine if you are motivated by positive or negative stimuli:

1. You would like to lose weight because:

    a. You'll feel better and have more energy.

    b. If you don't lose weight, you'll have to go on blood pressure medication.

2. You're staying late at work to finish an extra report because:

    a. You know your boss is thinking about giving you a raise, and you believe if you put in some extra time it might help your case.

    b. If you don't finish the extra report, that guy down the hall might do it and make you look bad.

3. You bought your spouse something they'd been wanting for a long time just as a surprise because:

    a. You love him or her and believe that one way you can show that love is through thoughtful gifts.

    b. You hate wasting money on dumb gifts, but you're afraid if you don't get the thing they want, they'll buy it anyway and you might as well get whatever points you can while you can.

4. You started taking a multivitamin because:

    a. You believe it will help support your health.

    b. You don't much care for vitamins, but you're afraid you might get sick if you don't take them.

5. You get annual checkups because:

    a. You want to make sure you're as healthy as you think you are and catch any small problems before they become big problems.

    b. You're afraid if you don't get checkups, you might suddenly have a heart attack and die.

6. You exercise three times a week because:

    a. It helps maintain your weight and strength.

    b. You hate exercise, but your spouse yells at you if you skip it, so what the heck … you do it.

7. You go to bed at the same time every night because:

    a. You know that a regular bedtime helps you to get a good night's sleep.

    b. If you didn't, you might fall asleep at work and lose your job.

If you have mostly A's, you are motivated by anticipation of positive outcomes. If you have mostly B's, you are motivated by fear of negative outcomes. Remember, these are just two different styles. One sort of person is not inherently "better" than the other. This information is intended simply to help you understand your motivational style so you can develop routines that will work for you.

If You See It, You Can Do It

Every single thing we see around us, from our cars to our hair dryers, stoves, and television sets, even our subdivisions, bridges, and apartment buildings, started as a glimmer in someone's mind. Imagination. Visualization. These are the fuels that power our dreams.

Imagination is so powerful it can actually define or constrain our behavior. Think of a child who believes there is a monster lurking under her bed at night. Once it gets dark, she will not get out of that bed for any reason because her imagined fear keeps her a prisoner there. But just as imagination can be a negative and paralyzing force in our lives, it can also be positive and energizing force. It all depends upon how we use it.

If you dream of living the wellness lifestyle, enjoying vibrant good health in a body that is strong and reliable, you are using the power of your imagination to create a new reality for yourself. And what is the bridge between your dreams and successful reality? Motivation. But we cannot get motivated before we have first defined our dreams and goals, and that is where visualization comes into play.

The Paintbox in Your Mind

If you truly desire to make permanent changes in your life, you must first change the way you think and behave. The idea of using creative visualization to create a new reality has been around for a long time, but a lot of people have dismissed it as so much hokum. Modern researchers have shown that using visualization to imagine desired outcomes can be very powerful.

All of us use visualization to some extent every day. As you lie in bed in the morning, perhaps you are trying to decide whether to wear your brown suit or navy pinstripe to an important meeting. As you think about it, you may unconsciously picture yourself in each suit, assess how each picture makes you feel, and determine your suit selection all in a matter of seconds, all based on subconscious deliberations you may not even have been fully aware of. All you know is that you suddenly got up out of bed, walked to your closet, and took out the navy pinstripe.

When you have a dream, you can use the paintbox of your imagination to color in all the details. You create an idea or mental image of your desired outcome. As you continue to focus on that idea or image, your energy and positive focus has a way of making that dream become a reality.

There are many ways to use creative visualization. Let's say you want to lose two dress or waist sizes before your birthday, which is four months away. You may start by seeing yourself as trim, but to ensure success, you should visualize yourself going through the steps necessary to achieve your goal. You might see yourself on a treadmill, lifting weights, or choosing healthy foods at a grocery store. And you might also want to visualize your reward, trying on the beautiful new dress or trim pair of pants. By imaging the desired outcome from start to finish and all the steps in between, you have essentially issued a set of instructions to your subconscious to tell it how to make your desires become reality.

Negative Visualization

You may not think that any phrase that has the word *negative* in it can be very good, but for some people, negative visualization, or fear of a certain outcome, can help them achieve their desires.

For example, let's say you have a competitor in an intraoffice race for a promotion. If fear of negative outcomes is what motivates you, you can visualize what it would feel like to let your competitor win the coveted job, and those feelings may be what spurs you on to higher performance and success.

You do need to be careful when using negative visualization to not let your fear level get out of hand or you may derail your own initiative. Don't let negativity slip into self-defeat.

Sometimes negative motivation can become so powerful that it paralyzes you. At that point, fear of negative outcomes no longer has any power to motivate you because the fear itself has become so all-encompassing that you can no longer act. If you feel like your fear has you stuck in a less than desirable place, you might want to seek assistance from a lifestyle coach or even get counseling to help you get past your fears and negativity. Although negativity isn't automatically a bad trait, if you let it dominate every facet of your life you'll be missing out on a lot.

Get Yourself a Wellness Partner

No one of us is perfect. We each have our little foibles and flaws. If you are having trouble sticking to a wellness program, you might want to consider enlisting a partner. It could be your spouse, your sibling, your best friend, or a neighbor. Tackling your wellness objectives with a partner can have multiple benefits for each of you. To begin with, you are much more likely to stick to a program if you have a partner working with you. You might feel a heightened sense of obligation to hold up a bargain if you are working with a partner. Having a wellness partner also helps to foster a sense of camaraderie and teamwork as you tackle and meet your wellness challenges. Finally, it gives you someone to help you over the rough spots, to encourage you when you feel down, and someone with whom you can celebrate your ultimate success.

The Least You Need to Know

◆ Before you start any wellness program, you should first figure out whether you are motivated more by positive or negative consequences.

◆ Creating a mission statement can help you stick to your goals.

◆ If you haven't ever experienced a "triggering event," you might not yet be motivated enough to stick to a wellness program.

◆ You can use the power of visualization to help make your dreams come true.

Chapter 26

Get Focused and Get Going

In This Chapter

- ◆ Now that you know everything …
- ◆ Switching to maintenance mode
- ◆ No more excuses
- ◆ Building self-confidence
- ◆ Reaping the rewards

Well, here we are at the end of our journey. We've given you a good overview of what it takes to live the wellness lifestyle and pointed you in many interesting directions. You have probably read things that appealed to you and made sense and things you thought were crazy or dumb. Now, you have to decide if wellness is something you truly want. And do you want it enough to adopt the changes necessary to make it part of your everyday life? We're hoping that you will.

In this last chapter, we'll give you some final bits of wisdom to help you get started with your wellness program and advice about what to do once you reach your goals. So get going! The rest is up to you.

Where to Begin

As we mentioned in the beginning of this book, it's not a good idea to tackle every single thing you want to change about your life all at once. If you know you have nutritional, exercise, and stress management issues, trying to fix them all at the same time will only lead to more stress and perhaps even failure. The last thing we want is for you to become discouraged before you even get started.

As you leaf back through this book, highlight sections that seem particularly appealing to you. Figure out the steps required to incorporate that behavior into your life on a regular basis and write them down. Talk to friends who have successfully made wellness part of their lifestyles and see if you can pick their brains for a few good, workable ideas. Ask them what sort of nutritional plan they follow, whether they exercise at home or in a gym, and how they manage their stress. Decide if you think what works for them will work for you.

Personalize Your Program

You may incorporate ideas from as many sources as necessary to make yourself a personalized game plan. Use what you have learned about yourself over the course of reading this book to make your program attractive and workable. If you put something in just because you think you have to but you really have no interest in doing it, then guess what? You're not going to do it. Don't add walking on a treadmill just because someone tells you you have to. If treadmills seem boring and dumb to you when you started reading this book, they probably still seem boring and dumb to you. The point is to build your program from elements that appeal to you. If you like bicycles, forget the treadmill. You can get the same aerobic benefit from a stationary bike with the additional bonus that you will be much more likely to perform an exercise you like that appeals to you than one you think is dumb.

Time Is of the Essence

Finally, be sure to anchor your goals to a timetable. If you don't, if you just hang your ideas out there without the defining framework of time, you are giving yourself a perfect excuse to never actually start your program. There will always be a tomorrow or a next week when you intend to get started, and if you don't say when that tomorrow is, it will never come.

For example, it is reasonable to expect to lose from 1 to 2 pounds a week, so if you have 40 pounds to lose, you know that will take you 20 to 40 weeks or 5 to 10 months to accomplish that goal. Remember to stay away from fad diets and pills and chose a nutritional plan that lets you select from a wide variety of healthful foods so you won't get bored. And remember, you are not dieting. You are following a nutritional plan that will enhance your health and help you lose weight at the same time.

If you are incorporating exercise into your schedule, don't try to go out and do three advanced aerobics classes and a weight training circuit on your first day—not unless you feel like spending the night in traction. Don't buy a $1,000 home gym or a $500 smoothie machine unless you know for certain that you will use them.

Start slowly. Buy or rent a beginner's aerobic videotape or enroll in a beginner's yoga class, and start there. If you can only make it through 5 or 10 minutes of the class, so what? At least you are trying. If you give up now you'll end up right back where you started—in the recliner with your remote control. But if you keep on going, within a couple of weeks you'll be able to manage 15 or 20 minutes of exercise at a time, and within a couple of months, you'll be able to breeze through the whole class with no difficulty at all.

> **Health Notes**
>
> The great Chinese philosopher Confucius probably never did aerobics or went on a diet, but nonetheless, he had something to say that can serve as an inspiration to anyone who is trying to reach a goal: "It does not matter how slowly you go as long as you do not stop." Just keep going, no matter how slowly, and you will eventually reach your goals.

Keep Raising Your Goals

As you conquer one goal, be sure to set another one. For example, if your goal was to get through an entire exercise video without stopping or getting overly tired, and you made that goal in three months, don't stop there. Go out and buy or rent an intermediate level tape, or enroll in a slightly more difficult class and challenge yourself to get through that.

If your goal was to walk one mile three days a week at three miles per hour, and it takes you two months to reach that goal, make your new goal to walk two miles at three miles per hour. When you have conquered a three-mile walk, try adding a day to your schedule so that you are walking on four days. If your schedule is tight, take a half-hour walk on busy days, and save the longer walks for days when you are less booked. Keep raising your goals as you reach new fitness levels in order to keep accruing fitness benefits.

Why is it necessary to keep setting your goals higher and higher? Because if your body reaches a certain level of fitness and you never challenge it beyond that level, your health and fitness improvements will stall there. You will never improve beyond that point. If you have 50 pounds to lose, you might lose the first 20 very quickly and then go weeks without seeing any additional loss if you never change your exercise routine. The same program that was incredibly tough when you started is not enough to challenge your new and fitter body. To keep the improvements coming, keep raising your goals.

In the same way, if one of your original goals was to cut back from five sodas a day to four, and you have successfully reached that goal, now try cutting back to three. When that feels comfortable, cut back to two, one, or maybe even none. Just remind yourself of all the empty calories that soda contains and how much weight you will lose simply by eliminating all those grams of sugar.

You can take this approach with any part of your wellness program. As long as you keep challenging yourself with new goals, you will continue to improve. The day you decide you're content with how things are is the day you will stop improving. Of course, if you have reached your ultimate goals, then that will be a pretty special day!

You've Reached Your Goals! Now What?

You're back in your old clothes, your blood pressure is down, you have energy to burn, and you feel like you're king or queen of the world. You're eating a great diet, and stress doesn't get to you the way it used to. You're sleeping soundly every night and have a bounce in your step, and all your friends and co-workers are asking you what in the world you've been doing.

Congratulations! Once you've reached all your wellness goals, you might be tempted just to sit back and celebrate your success. Maybe a giant chunk of cheesecake sounds good, or maybe you think you should pay yourself back for all the hours you've put in at the gym, so you're just going to let yourself skip this one week, just this one. And there's a great movie on from midnight until 2 A.M., and your VCR isn't working, so you're just going to stay up late tonight, eat your cheesecake, watch the midnight movie, and not exercise. Just for tonight.

The only trouble with this approach is that if you sit around and celebrate for too long, pretty soon you'll be right back where you started. And you don't want all your hard work to go to waste, do you?

Confine your celebration to something reasonable. A small slice of cheesecake, a day off from the gym instead of a week off, and to heck with the late movie. Your body needs its sleep, and you can always watch a movie later, VCR or no VCR. Make a conscious effort to put your wellness needs first until it becomes a habit. Use that priority to help you make tough decisions, and you won't ever go wrong.

Maintenance Mode

Once you have reached your wellness goals, you can ease into a maintenance mode. When you switch to maintenance, you'll find that you don't have to work quite as hard to maintain the results you've achieved over the initial phase of your wellness program.

Let's say you had worked your way up to walking an hour a day five days a week. When you reach your goals, you might find that you can maintain your fitness level even if you cut back to walking just three days a week, or keep the five-day schedule but cut back to a half-hour walk. You will have to experiment a bit to see what works best for you. If you cut back and start to gain weight or feel sluggish, then obviously you have cut back too much. And there's no rule saying you absolutely have to cut back once you reach your goals; you may be so happy with your results that you want to remain indefinitely on the program that helped you achieve your success.

Eat a Little More

Using the same line of thinking, you may want to be a bit more generous with your meal portions once you reach your goal weight. If you've been eating four ounces of lean protein at dinner, try raising that to five ounces and see what happens. Add a small treat a couple of times a week, like a piece of fine chocolate or a glass of good wine. Your body will tell you if what you are doing is okay.

If you continue to maintain your results even after you have increased portion size and added a few weekly treats, then you'll know your body is utilizing the larger portions without difficulty. If you start to gain weight, however, you'll know that the increase in portion sizes is more than what your body can handle.

Of course, we hope you're not going to go hog wild and jump right back into all those old, detrimental eating habits that got you in trouble in the first place. Don't go scarfing down a whole bag of greasy potato chips to celebrate your success. You're over that. Remember? Everybody can stand a little treat now and then, just make sure the treats don't lead you down the path of temptation past the point where you can resist their siren call. Remember what we've said right from the beginning of this book: moderation, not deprivation.

Let that be your guiding mantra as you begin to reincorporate some food items into your nutritional plan that you avoided during the initial phase of your program. One thing that might surprise you is that some things you used to think were downright delicious might not taste so good to you anymore. This is particularly true of sticky-sweet sodas, candies, and greasy snacks like chips and puffs.

If you go a long time without eating any of these junk foods and then try them again, you might find that their taste seems artificial and yucky. It happens to everyone who remakes their eating habits. Once they get used to the taste of fresh, natural food, the junky stuff just doesn't seem appealing any more. In fact, it might seem downright repulsive.

You Mean You Haven't Started?

Perhaps you've read this far and still haven't decided whether or not to embark on a fitness program. What are you waiting for? We've heard all the possible excuses, so don't even go there. You will always be able to come up with a justification for not starting, some of them quite reasonable. But the point is, this is "No More Excuses!" time. Stop spending so much energy trying to figure out reasons why you are not on a wellness program and devote that same energy to getting with a program. It doesn't matter which one you choose; it only matters that you get started and stick with it.

"No More Excuses!"

We don't care how creative you are, there is not a single excuse you can think up to explain why you are not going on a wellness program. None of them will hold water.

From the Medicine Chest _____

Top Ten Reasons for Not Embarking on a Wellness Program

10. A meteor landed on the hood of my car.

9. I was going to the gym but got abducted by aliens.

8. My cat had kittens on my treadmill.

7. My mother-in-law gets offended if I don't eat her lasagna.

6. I really like being sick all the time.

5. It's against my religion.

4. I'd rather just have the surgery.

3. Chocolate is my life.

2. I thr-thr-thr-thrive on stress. Da-don't you?

… and the number one reason for not embarking on a wellness program is (drum roll, please) …

1. I turned my stair-stepper into an Art Deco clothes hanger, and the Museum of Modern Art just paid me a million dollars for it and took it away.

Okay, so maybe these reasons are slightly bogus, but they're at least as good as anything you can come up with, right?

The point is you can make up excuses for not getting started from now until doomsday, but they will still be just that—excuses. And the more excuses you give yourself and the longer you wait until you get started, the longer it will be before you see results. And if you're really good at making up excuses, you might never get started. And you don't want that to happen, do you?

Change Your Self Talk

Another exercise you might want to try is to change the way you talk to yourself. The next time you hear yourself making some excuse about not watching your nutrition or not exercising, stop yourself and say, "I am going to start my wellness plan today at lunch. I will order bottled water instead of soda and a salad instead of a cheeseburger." And just like that you will have gotten started.

In the beginning you may start and stop many times over. Just keep going, just keep starting and like the stubborn engine on the lawnmower that's been sitting in the shed all winter, one day your determination will roar to life and you will be off and running. Quit telling yourself you can't do it, and start telling yourself you can, and one day you actually will.

Believe in Yourself

Maybe you are hesitating because you still haven't quite convinced yourself that you deserve all this extra effort and attention. After all, there are so many other people depending on you, how can you possibly take time to do all these wellness activities for yourself?

Remember what we told you back in Chapter 24, "You Deserve It—Convincing Yourself That Wellness Is Important," that self-sacrifice is fine up to a point, but after that point it becomes self-destructive. What is needed here is another "self" word, and that word is "self-confidence." Do whatever it takes to convince yourself to get started on a wellness program, then watch your self-confidence grow. The people you love, the people who depend on you, will watch in amazement, too, as your success in achieving your wellness goals filters out into every other aspect of your life and builds your self-confidence.

If you have successfully completed your wellness program and achieved the goals you set for yourself, you are already enjoying your biggest and best reward—the renewed health and vigor that such a program brings. But there are other rewards as well, and you'll soon start discovering them.

We live in a culture where fit people are almost revered. People look at you and know the amount of work it takes to maintain a fit body, and they automatically start making some assumptions about the sort of person who cares enough to take such good care of themselves. Unless there's a jealousy factor at work, those assumptions are generally pretty good.

They will think that you are disciplined (and you are), hard-working, goal-oriented, a closer or someone who finishes what they start, persistent, strong-willed, determined, and lots of other good things.

Being fit will help you in other areas of your life as well. Whether you are single or married, your significant other is sure to appreciate the brand-new you. If you don't happen to have a partner, your trim new look will surely help you attract one.

You will also look better in your clothes, and if you have gone from a large size to a standard size, you'll suddenly discover that the selection and variety of styles available to you has increased exponentially.

You'll feel better about yourself and more in control of your life and your health. Your stress-management skills will help shield you from the sort of upsets that used to derail you. You'll know how to handle problems while they are still small.

Best of all, instead of avoiding your health issues, you will now have the confidence and knowledge you need to address health problems as they arise.

The Least You Need to Know

- ◆ Anchor your wellness program to a timetable.
- ◆ As you reach certain levels of achievement, keep raising your goals to keep improving.
- ◆ Once you reach your wellness goals, you can maintain your results by switching over to a less-strenuous program.
- ◆ If you keep making excuses about why you can't start a wellness program, you never will start.
- ◆ To build your self-confidence, change your self talk.

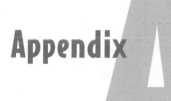

Appendix A

Resources

The Internet has become a wonderful source for information relating to health, fitness, nutrition, and wellness. In fact, there is so much available that it's sometimes difficult to distinguish between the good and not-so-good when surfing the Net.

We've done some surfing for you and recommend the following sites as good sources of information for many of the topics covered in this book.

The following sites contain good general information about health and wellness:

WebMD.com
www.webmd.com
Geared toward the consumer, WebMD.com contains an excellent overview of the most common health complaints under "Condition Center," along with some savvy tips for dealing with the problem. It also features special sections for pregnancy, staying healthy, and living with a chronic illness.

Centers for Disease Control
www.cdc.gov
The U.S. government funds the Centers for Disease Control, located in Atlanta. CDC monitors disease outbreaks such as flu and meningitis and issues health alerts and consumer advisories. There is a lot of good information on this site.

National Institutes of Health
www.nih.gov
NIH is another governmental agency, charged with the responsibility to disseminate current health information and news about ongoing studies and

clinical trials. It also contains information about more than 9,000 different prescription drugs and toll-free numbers where consumers can get information about a variety of health conditions.

Kaiser Permanente

www.kaiserpermanente.org/toyourhealth

This website of one of the most famous health-care providers in America provides good topical health information. Here you will meet Dr. Sidney Garfield, the innovative doctor who, in 1933, established the first prepaid health plan for workers on the Los Angeles Aqueduct. All modern HMOs and PPOs spring from his example.

ThirdAge.com

www.thirdage.com

This site offers a variety of information on a wide range of topics relating to physical and emotional health.

ODPHP

www.odphp.osophs.dhhs.gov

The government's Office of Disease Prevention and Health Promotion offers news about Public Health and Science.

Mayo Clinic

www.mayo.edu/healthinfo/info.html

Easy-to-understand information about a variety of diseases and conditions with links to other web resources.

Healthy People Fact Sheet

odphp.osoph.dhhs.gov

Information about the government's Healthy People 2010 initiative.

Arnot Ogden Medical Center

www.aomc.org

General health-care information.

Department of Health and Human Services
Agency for Healthcare Research and Quality

www.ahrq.gov/clinic/uspstfix.htm

The experts on this site review clinical treatment protocols for effectiveness and make recommendations based on those evaluations.

Red Cross

www.redcross.org

The Red Cross provides news and information about a variety of topics, including disaster preparedness and first aid, among others.

Office of the Surgeon General

www.surgeongeneral.gov

This government-sponsored site offers up-to-date information on a variety of topics, including smoking cessation, suicide prevention, bioterrorism, and many others.

The following websites contain information relating to one or more particular diseases or health problems:

American Cancer Society

www.cancer.org

This site contains helpful information about cancer symptoms, diagnosis, and treatment options, along with links to patient and family support groups.

American Heart Association

www.americanheart.org

This site offers all the latest news and information about heart disease and strokes, including comprehensive information about symptoms, diagnosis, and treatment.

National Institute of Mental Health

www.mhsource.com

Contains information about a wide variety of mental health issues and conditions, including breaking news.

National Kidney Foundation

www.kidney.org

Directed at patients who are suffering from kidney disease, this site contains information on everything from dialysis to transplants.

National Institute of Diabetes and Digestive and Kidney Diseases

www.niddk.nih.gov

Sponsored by the U.S. government, this informative site contains a vast storehouse of information on diverse topics relating to diabetes, obesity, and kidney disease.

National Heart, Lung and Blood Institute

www.nhlbi.nih.gov

This government-sponsored site offers informative articles on cardiovascular and pulmonary disease.

American Diabetes Association

www.diabetes.org

This site contains useful information about the diagnosis and treatment of diabetes, along with symptoms to watch for and links to patient support organizations.

Arthritis Foundation

www.arthritis.org

Information and patient support for victims of arthritis.

The following websites contain information on exercise and fitness:

American Council on Exercise
www.acefitness.org
Tips on exercise and information for people who would like to work in the fitness field.

YMCA (Young Men's Christian Association)
www.ymca.com/find_your_y/findy_nav.htm
Find your local YMCA.

The following websites offer information about stress:

prcn.org/next/stress.html
Predict your chance of experiencing an illness or accident within the upcoming two years based on your stress level.

stress.about.com/cs/supportsystems/
Find an online stress management support group.

The following websites offer information about nutrition, grocery shopping, and related topics:

www.culligan.com/athome-h2o-calc.asp
Calculate your daily water requirements.

wwww.crnusa.org/Shellscire000002.html
A comparison of RDAs, RDIs, and DRIs for vitamins and minerals.

www.thefrugalshopper.com/tips/grshopping.html
A complete list of smart tips to help you save time and money at the grocery.

www.dhl-usa.com/lbs-2-kilo
Calculate your body's protein requirements.

www.usda.gov/news/releases/2001/01/whitepaperexe.htm
Compare the pros and cons of various diets.

www.eatright.org
Find a registered dietitian in your community.

The following websites offer nutritious and appealing meals that can be prepared quickly:

www.allrecipes.com

www.ivillage.com/food/recipefinder

www.recipeland.com

www.my-meals.com

Glossary

action   The period of time during which you begin to do whatever is necessary to make change.

acupressure   The ancient Chinese practice of applying pressure on specific points on the body for therapeutic purposes.

acupuncture   The ancient Chinese practice of inserting very fine needles into specific points on the skin for therapeutic purposes. Western doctors were amazed when they first observed Chinese surgeons performing surgery using no anesthesia other than carefully placed acupuncture needles.

aerobic capacity   The ability of your muscles to absorb oxygen for use as fuel.

aerobic exercise   Any exercise that requires your heart and lungs to work harder to supply a sufficient amount of oxygen to your muscles.

allopathic medicine   Allopathic medicine is practiced by licensed medical doctors and governed by the American Medical Association and state boards. It focuses on the physical causes of illness and rarely deals with a mind-spirit connection. Allopathic medicine is known for its high percentage of accurate diagnoses and swift and effective treatment to alleviate traumatic injuries and sudden illnesses.

allopathic training   A course of mainstream medical training that culminates with the conferring of the degree of M.D., or medical doctor.

anaerobic exercise   The word *anaerobic* literally means "without oxygen." Anaerobic exercise is any exercise that uses oxygen more quickly than your body can supply it, like weight training. Because your body tires rapidly during anaerobic exercise, it requires rest periods between periods of exercise to replenish its energy.

analgesic   Any medication or device that relieves pain without inducing loss of consciousness.

angina   Brief, spasmodic attacks of intense chest pain caused by insufficient oxygenation of the heart muscle.

anthelmintic   Any agent that expels parasites from the body, especially intestinal parasites.

antibiotic   A class of drugs designed to combat bacterial infections. The word means literally "against life," because antibiotics were intended to kill or destroy disease-causing organisms.

antioxidant   Any substance that inhibits oxidation, or the oxidizing effects of oxygen, including hardening of the arteries.

antipyretic   Any agent that reduces fever.

antiseptic   A substance, usually applied topically, that inhibits the growth of bacteria that may cause infections.

apoptosis   A biological regulatory mechanism through which damaged, old, or rogue cells kill themselves off in an orderly fashion, thereby maintaining a desirable state of homeostasis in the body. Also called PCD, or programmed cell death.

atherosclerosis   A hardening of the arteries characterized by deposits of plaque and fibrous tissues on and within the walls of arteries.

basal metabolic rate   The amount of energy your body requires every day to perform its most basic functions like breathing, digesting your food, and circulating blood throughout your body.

body mass index or BMI   Your weight in kilograms divided by your height in meters, squared. A BMI between 19 and 24 is considered healthy, a BMI of 25 or more is considered overweight, and a BMI of 30 or greater is considered morbidly obese.

bone density   The strength or density of your bones.

bruxism   The habit of grinding the teeth together, often related to stress or a nervous condition.

burnout   The exhaustion of physical and emotional strength accompanied by a near-total lack of motivation that usually results from prolonged stress or frustration.

carcinogens   An agent or substance that may trigger the onset of cancer.

cardiomyopathy   A chronic heart condition characterized by damage to the heart muscle and overgrowth of cardiac muscle fibers, resulting in a weakened heart that cannot perform its job properly.

chi   According to Traditional Chinese Medical practitioners, the chi is the energy flow or life force of the body.

circadian rhythms   Cycles of biological activity and behavior that occur within a 24-hour period that are generated by an internal clock synchronized to light-dark cycles in the environment.

cognitive dissonance   When someone's beliefs and behavior are inconsistent, they are suffering from cognitive dissonance.

contemplation stage   The period during which you really start to think about making a change.

CPT   Certified Personal Trainer, a designation awarded by several national fitness associations to trainers who have successfully completed a specific course of study.

diastole   The term used to describe the dilation of the heart during the time it fills with blood in between the contractions or beats that pump blood out to the body.

distress   The emotion triggered by any negative event or feeling. If present over a long period of time, distress can have severe negative consequences on physical health.

diuretic   Any substance that increases the flow of urine.

electrolytes   Nonmetallic electrical conductors that convey electrical signals through the movement of ions.

endorphin   A form of morphine produced naturally in the body.

essential fatty acids   Omega 3, Omega 6, and Omega 9; lipids that are essential to the proper functioning of the body. They are called essential because we cannot manufacture them in our bodies and must get our requirements from the food we eat.

eustress   The pleasurable emotion that accompanies feelings of success, fulfillment, and accomplishment.

fiber   The indigestible portion of our food, fiber is vital to stimulate peristalsis or movement of the intestines.

folic acid   An essential water-soluble vitamin that is a member of the B-vitamin family. Also called vitamin B-9.

free radical   Unstable compounds produced when the body burns fuel for energy, free radicals cause cell damage that has been linked with aging and the onset of several diseases associated with aging like arthritis and osteoporosis. May be offset by consumption of sufficient antioxidants like beta-carotene.

glycemic index   The measure of how rapidly a food is digested and how quickly its sugar content gets into the bloodstream.

glycogen   Glycogen is glucose in storage form in the liver.

H$_2$0   The chemical symbol for water.

heat exhaustion   Heat exhaustion occurs when people exercise heavily or work in a hot, humid atmosphere. Blood flow to the skin increases, causing blood flow to decrease to the vital organs, resulting in mild shock. Heavy sweating causes dehydration and a loss of electrolytes, which can upset the body's delicate electrical system. If not treated, heat exhaustion can quickly progress to heat stroke, a life-threatening medical emergency.

heat stroke   A life-threatening condition. Occurs when the victim's temperature control system, which produces sweating to cool the body, stops working. The body temperature can rise so high that brain damage and death may result if the body is not cooled quickly.

holistic   Concerned with the treatment of complete systems rather than the analysis or treatment of separate parts. For example, holistic health-care practitioners believe it is necessary to consider the entire patient—mind, body, and spirit—in order to achieve the most effective treatment of any illness or injury.

homeostasis   A relatively stable state of equilibrium or a tendency toward such a state between the different but interdependent elements or groups of elements of an organism, population, or group.

hypertension   High blood pressure. Any value below 120 over 80 is considered normal blood pressure, 135 over 90 is high normal, and anything above 140 over 90 is high blood pressure or hypertension.

insomnia   The prolonged and usually abnormal inability to obtain adequate sleep.

junk food   Food that is high in calories but low in nutritional content.

ketosis   A condition produced by an abnormal increase in ketones in the body, brought about by starvation or uncontrolled diabetes.

lipids   Any of various substances that includes fats, waxes, and related compounds that, with proteins and carbohydrates, constitute the principal structural components of living cells.

maintenance   The period after you have reached a goal, during which you find a new identity and work to avoid lapses in your behavior that might undermine your new identity.

motivation   The reason behind why you take an action; the bridge between an idea and its fruition. Motivation makes you put ideas into action. If you have motivation, you act because you want to, not because you have to.

phytonutrients   Plant-derived components that have exhibited either nutritive or metabolic biological activity.

precontemplation   The period of time when you become aware and start to really pay attention to a problem.

preparation   The period of time during which you begin to form a game plan to address a particular problem.

progressive relaxation   Introduced in 1935, progressive relaxation is a well-accepted stress reduction technique that involves alternately tensing and relaxing muscles.

RDA   Recommended Dietary Allowance. The 1968 U.S. Department of Agriculture standards for minimal intakes of certain vitamins and minerals required to maintain health. There has been a certain amount of controversy since the USDA switched to RDI or Reference Daily Intake standard. Even though RDIs are based on the 1968 RDA recommendations, they do not take into account age and gender differences, and many dietitians argue they are not as safe or accurate as a result.

RDI   Reference Daily Intake. *See* RDA.

resistance training   A method of conditioning designed to increase muscle strength, endurance, and power.

reticular activating system   The reticular activating system functions as a communication link between the mind and the body. For example, writing things down makes them concrete in a way that just imagining and thinking about them doesn't.

The Sedona Method   A stress-reduction technique introduced in 1974 that teaches people to let go of negative emotions and develop a more positive outlook on life.

shiatsu   A form of massage that uses pressure from fingers, thumbs, and sometimes elbows, knees, hands, and feet applied to acupuncture points and meridians to stimulate the flow of energy.

sleep deficit   The difference between the number of hours of sleep you need and the number of hours you actually get.

super bug   Any bacterial organism that has, through repeated overexposure to antibiotics, mutated and grown resistant to standard antibiotic treatment.

systole   Describes the heart contraction that forces blood out to circulate through the lungs for oxygenation prior to circulating throughout the body.

tai chi   An ancient Chinese discipline that involves slow, deliberate movements to stretch and condition muscles.

TCM (Traditional Chinese Medicine)   Aims to restore and maintain the energy balance in the chi, or life force of the body. Practitioners believe illness results from stagnation in the flow of chi in the body, which prevents the body from draining fluids as it should. TCM includes acupuncture, herbal treatment, dietary therapy, and exercise.

trigger   A subconscious response to external or internal stimuli, resulting in a predictable behavior.

wellness   A condition of excellent physical and mental health actively maintained through a sound program of good nutrition, moderate regular exercise, stress management, and preventive maintenance.

Index

D

E

F

G

H

I

S

T

U

X-Z